A MINUTE *for* Caregivers

When Every Day Feels Like Monday

PETER ROSENBERGER

FIDELIS
PUBLISHING

FIDELIS PUBLISHING *

ISBN: 9781956454307 /
ISBN: 9781956454314 (eBook)

A Minute for Caregivers: When Every Day Feels Like Monday
© 2023 Peter W. Rosenberger

Cover Design by Diana Lawrence
Interior Layout by Lisa Parnell
Edited by Amanda Varian

Scripture quotations marked ESV are from The ESV® Bible (The Holy Bible, English Standard Version®), copyright © 2001 by Crossway, a publishing ministry of Good News Publishers. Used by permission. All rights reserved.

Scripture quotations marked NIV are taken from THE HOLY BIBLE, NEW INTERNATIONAL VERSION®, NIV® Copyright © 1973, 1978, 1984, 2011 by Biblica, Inc.® Used by permission. All rights reserved worldwide.

Scripture quotations marked NKJV are from the New King James Version®. Copyright © 1982 by Thomas Nelson. Used by permission. All rights reserved.

Scripture marked MSG is from *The Message*, copyright © 1993, 2002, 2018 by Eugene H. Peterson. Used by permission of NavPress. All rights reserved. Represented by Tyndale House Publishers.

Scripture marked KJV is from the King James Version. Public Domain.

Order at www.faithfultext.com for a significant discount. Email info@fidelispublishing.com to inquire about bulk purchase discounts.

Fidelis Publishing, LLC Sterling, VA • Nashville, TN - fidelispublishing.com

Manufactured in the United States of America

10 9 8 7 6 5 4 3 2 1

Foreword by Oliver L. North

· · · · ·

The Mayo Clinic diagnosis wasn't good—but at least we had one, instead of guessing. After returning from an assignment as an embedded correspondent and host of *War Stories* on FOX News, I believed Betsy—the half-century-plus love of my life; my best friend on earth; mom to our four magnificent adult children; "Nan" to our eighteen terrific grandchildren—must have had a stroke. Lots of people, including my own mother, recovered from strokes. *Betsy will too*, I hoped. I was wrong.

After several days of carefully examining Betsy and countless images of her head and body, the extraordinary doctors at Mayo gently delivered their findings—verbally and in writing: "Your wife has a degenerative, asymmetric brain disorder called corticobasal syndrome . . . It is characterized by apraxia and rigidity on one side of the body . . . These symptoms are often accompanied by dementia and 'cognitive disarray' . . . As of now, it is incurable, and untreatable . . ."

My initial reaction to this devastating diagnosis was, *Betsy, you and I have been through a lot together. We have so many things planned for our "Golden Years"! I'm a U.S. Marine; we're a team and followers of the Miracle Worker, Jesus Christ! We're going to beat this evil malady.* But we haven't.

Shortly after we returned home from Rochester, Minnesota, MajGen John Grinalds, USMC (Ret) and his wife, Norwood—dear friends since the 1970s when their examples led us to our faith in Christ—came to visit us. After listening to the diagnosis, John asked, "Who are you feeling sorry for, Betsy or you?"

After thinking about it, I replied, "Me."

John nodded and said, "Your new mission, Marine, is become the very best caregiver Betsy will ever have on earth!"

Thus, began for me, the most challenging physical, mental, emotional, and spiritual experience of my eighty years on earth. That was nearly five years ago.

Despite many months of reading, listening to "coaches," viewing countless videos, even keeping company with several thousand terribly wounded Soldiers, Sailors, Airmen, Guardsmen, and Marines—and their families—I was exhausted and adrift on how to be Betsy's caregiver.

Then, Peter Rosenberger sent his draft of this inspiring book. *Finally*, I thought, *someone who knows what I'm going through. He's been there, done that!*

A Minute for Caregivers is now my "go-to" primer for every challenge I face in caring for my best friend. If being a caregiver to someone you love is part of your life, you need this book.

Introduction

· · · · ·

"I'd recommend a book for you to read,
but *you're* the guy to write it!"

Walking into a mental health facility in Nashville, I stood silently for a moment until a woman at the front desk asked, "Are you lost?"

With tears filling my eyes, I nodded while muttering, "I guess I am."

Sniffling a bit, I wryly asked, "Do you all take walk-ins?"

Both people sitting behind the counter responded with strange looks on their faces.

With exasperation, I inwardly asked, *Really?! This is a mental health facility, and that's the question that gets me a funny look? It's not like I was dressed as a Wookie or anything!*

"Would you like to talk to a counselor?"

Prudently holding my tongue while nodding affirmatively, I followed them to another counter. After staff members took my wallet, keys, and later my blood pressure, I found myself at a dilapidated table in a stark room. With faded paint on the walls and chairs that had seen better days, I felt like I sat in a precinct interrogation room from what can best be described as "early *Law and Order*." After a few minutes, a pleasant woman opened the door and introduced herself as a staff counselor.

"What's brought you here today, Peter?"

Haltingly, I recounted the journey of my life as a family caregiver. Many years into the role by that time, I also shared my own recent surgery that went sideways—nearly causing me to bleed out on the table. Four units of blood, a post-op infection, and a bumpy recovery later, I discovered the inability to sleep. Simply put, I felt spent.

It all tumbled out to this patient woman. I dumped a lifetime's supply of frustration, weariness, resentment, fear, obligation, guilt, shame, heartache, and anger onto the battered table. But behind all those feelings lay the even greater anguish of grief.

Such is the life of a family caregiver.

To date, my wife, Gracie, has endured more than eighty-five operations, including the amputation of both legs. More than 100 physicians have treated her in thirteen hospitals. In addition, Gracie has undergone 150+ minor procedures and lives with relentless pain—all from a 1983 car accident when she was only seventeen. I met her a few years after her ordeal following surgery #21. She lost her legs after our children were born, and although we experienced seasons without massive trials, those seasons remained short and infrequent.

Following my marathon purging in the "examination" room, I took a deep breath and waited for the counselor's response. The overpowering weariness and angst led me to hope I could stay and receive "treatment" for exhaustion. What I really wanted was rest.

It turns out they don't do that sort of thing (except maybe in Hollywood during the 1940s).

After telling a trained mental health professional that I felt I was crazy—while *inside* a mental health facility—I admit to experiencing great curiosity about what would happen next.

Thinking for a moment, she said, "You know I can't keep you here."

"You're not crazy," she quickly added.

With a raised eyebrow, I asked if I could get that in writing.

"There's quite a list who'd like to see that," I muttered glumly.

Chuckling, she further said, "No, you're not crazy, but you are burned out."

Retrieving a notepad from her jacket, she wrote some names and offered, "I can refer you to some counselors who might be helpful."

Nodding in acceptance, I took her list. Switching gears, she added, "We've been giving out box lunches to people today, and there's one left. It's tuna fish—you want it?"

Not once have I turned down a tuna fish sandwich, and the record remains intact.

Escorting me out of the room, she led me across the hall and grabbed the last box lunch from the refrigerator. Handing it to me, she added something that would change my life.

"I'd recommend a book for you to read, but *you're* the guy to write it."

Reclaiming my wallet and keys, I trekked to the parking lot. Without turning the car on, I sat quietly behind the wheel and opened the box to see a sandwich, soda, chips, apple, and cookie. Savoring every bite as if from the finest restaurant, I reflected on her words about me writing a book for caregivers.

"What kind of book would I write for caregivers?" I scoffed to myself.

"What would I say to them?"

Taking another bite, I half snorted, "What would I say to myself?"

Those questions launched my journey into learning the language of caregivers.

Drawing upon my 35+ years (and counting) of caring for my wife, I've answered those questions and more. Now "fluent in caregiver," I speak directly to caregivers' hearts and address the train wreck behind the weary eyes of those who stand between a vulnerable loved one and an even worse disaster.

Sadly, I don't remember the name of that counselor who helped direct my feet to what would become my life's work. Yet I remain deeply grateful she saw past my distress and offered compassion, insights, and sustenance for the journey—even if it was just a box lunch.

The inspiration for this current book unexpectedly arrived while talking with an individual at a doctor's billing office. When I inquired how she was doing that day, she enthusiastically exclaimed, "Great . . . it's Friday!"

Without thinking, I (embarrassingly) grumbled, "Friday means nothing to me . . . every day is Monday."

After finishing that conversation, I considered the reality of "Every day is Monday"—not just for me, but for many of my fellow caregivers. Knowing the existence of the caregiving life, I sought to give myself and other caregivers a one-minute message to strengthen us for those "every day is Monday" moments.

The job of a family caregiver remains filled with "many dangers, toils, and snares." As a burned-out caregiver, I tried to have myself committed to a mental health institution, but all I received was a tuna sandwich—along with the invitation to dig deep within and help point fellow caregivers to safety, often for one minute at a time.

● ● ●

Resolve never to quit, never to give up,
no matter what the situation. —Jack Nicklaus

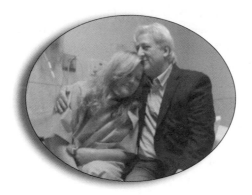

1

The Opinions of Others

· · · · ·

In 1986, my wife (then fiancé) underwent surgery on her right ankle to save her crushed leg. Although she ultimately lost both legs years later, hope remained in the driver's seat at the time. While this surgery was her 22nd (best count) since her 1983 car accident, it was my first with her. Following the operation, the surgeon provided a favorable report, and everyone expressed relief. Stating she'd be in recovery for some time, he suggested, "You can't see her for a while, so why don't you take a break."

Following "doctor's orders," I went to a movie.

I later learned of the clutched pearls and tongue-clucking that occurred while I sat in the theater. One of them, a holy-roller type with a *"My Other Car Is a Chariot of Fire"* bumper sticker on her Cadillac, piled onto Gracie's family about my inability to care for her.

Stunned at the response, I mistakenly allowed shame and fear of disapproval to drive future actions. That unfortunate pattern continued for years before learning to trust my instincts. I also better discovered how to handle unsolicited opinions flung by the ill-informed and inexperienced.

Trusting in our instincts while detaching from others' disapproval helps avoid resentment while allowing clarity of thought—and caregivers desperately need to think clearly. It's okay to watch a movie, go for a drive, take a walk, and by all means, keep firm boundaries with the "pearl clutchers"!

• • •

None are more unjust in their judgments
of others than those who have a high opinion
of themselves. —Charles Spurgeon

2

Collect the Facts and Fears

• • • • •

A listener shared her frustration, weariness, and burnout after years of caring for her husband following a traumatic brain injury. At sixty-eight, she expressed growing concern regarding her abilities—and his diminishing ones.

"He's got a colostomy, ileostomy, and a host of other physical issues requiring full-time care—and I'm just exhausted. His mind is sharp, but his body is severely impaired, and I'm conflicted about a long-term care facility."

Listening to her "get it all out," I shared: "It seems you're nearing a decision point where his needs eclipse your efforts; you may be closer than you realize. Regardless, how about writing down what an appropriate long-term facility looks like for you and your husband? With that in mind, and given the waiting lists for so many facilities, you can seek the proper place together while you can still care for him. If the crisis moment arrives, you've already paved the road so that the transition is a bit smoother."

As caregivers, we often must make decisions that benefit the whole unit—not just one person. The unit depends upon a capable caregiver, but fear, guilt, and obligation can hamper making the best possible decision in an impossible situation.

So many couples struggle with this dynamic, and there's no easy path. Wedding vows discuss long-term care but not long-term care facilities. Yet leaning on a facility doesn't equate to abandoning the vows; instead, it can help both parties better keep them.

• • •

When you have collected all the facts and
fears and made your decision, turn off all
your fears and go ahead! —George S. Patton

3

Aggressive Assurance

· · · · ·

During a recent medical event with my wife, she received significant time with the acute pain management team. To my surprise, they engaged me, asked questions, and solicited my thoughts as Gracie's longtime caregiver. Recognizing that post-operative pain management with her is a bit of a trick, they listened as I shared numerous "incidents" from her long journey.

After relating her history, I added, "In my experience, I've found that one of the most effective ways to help her is 'aggressive assurance.' Constantly reinforcing, 'We've got you—and we're on top of this.'"

The pain management professor immediately jumped in and addressed his students, "I can't agree more with the importance of assuring the patient—and easing the anxiety," he stated emphatically. "Chronic pain patients understand pain in ways we can't because they live with it daily. They also know what it's like to experience intractable pain and the terror involved when unable to communicate—or the frustration of not being understood."

The students, professor, and I talked a bit more, and I watched them scramble to take notes and remember the importance of aggressive assurance for patients in pain.

Later, the professor returned to the room and specifically asked to see me.

As he detailed the plan his team implemented to help Gracie, my eyes filled with tears when he looked at me and quietly said, "Caregivers also respond well to aggressive assurance."

● ● ●

From caring comes courage. —*Lao Tzu*

4

Do the Next Right Thing

• • • • •

If caregivers mapped out a decision tree for our daily lives, it would look like a forest. Each day we're faced with numerous choices—and most seem filled with unpleasant outcomes. Sometimes the decisions before us have a paralyzing effect, and we don't know what to do next.

In those moments, we serve ourselves well to choose the next right thing as our action step. The big problems become more approachable when our heads and hearts calm down.

For that to happen, our decisions require "reduction."

Unlike the giant single unpleasant task of "eating the elephant one bite at a time," decision reduction helps us focus by redirecting our eyes from the myriad choices to the micro-steps in our path. Maybe the next right thing is to drink water, sit down with a bowl of soup, take a nap, or even go for a walk. Although the problem usually remains, we tackle it better with a calmer and more disciplined mind.

When offered this path, we invariably know the next right thing to do; we just usually need permission—not from others but ourselves.

The Bible supports this when affirming that God's Word is "a lamp unto my feet."

It's a lamp, not a searchlight. Do the next right thing—with the light provided.

• • •

Not until we are lost do we
begin to understand ourselves.
—Henry David Thoreau

5

Harsh Judgment

* * * * *

Interviewing a couple who raised two children with Huntington's disease (HD) on my program, they relayed a heartbreaking story where they stood before a judge who clearly didn't understand the nature of HD. After repeated arrests for shoplifting, violent behavior, and other issues, the judge commented from the bench that she felt this resulted from "bad parenting." Unable to address the court or defend themselves, the couple shared, "We had to take it on the chin."

A five-minute search or phone call by the judge would have provided a bigger picture of the nature of this horrific disease that brutalizes both patients and their caregivers. Sadly, the judge chose to go with an uninformed decision—and a regrettable lack of compassion.

While the judge's comments remain grievous, how many caregivers "don the black robe" and make harsh and ill-informed pronouncements upon themselves while looking in the mirror? Countless caregivers spend way too much time condemning themselves for the out-of-control behavior of someone else. Whatever we wish that judge to have said to this broken and despairing couple, we would benefit from posting that same message on our bathroom mirrors.

• • •

I have always found that mercy
bears richer fruits than strict justice.
—Abraham Lincoln

6

Facing Our Giants

· · · · ·

Before the famous altercation with Goliath, when David expressed anger at the blasphemous giant, one of his embarrassed older brothers who camped at the battle scene furiously derided him. But King Saul heard about David, and astonishingly, the king allowed the teenager to fight Goliath. Saul even put his tunic and armor on him. Saul was tall, but David wasn't, and the king's armor didn't fit. Struggling to function in the ill-fitting battle garb, David removed it and faced Goliath his way—depending upon God's might. David recognized he couldn't succeed while wearing something that didn't fit him.

How many try to "conquer a Goliath" while wearing something that doesn't fit? The conditions of our loved ones serve as formidable giants to us, and we can't fight them while trying to be, do, and act like something that doesn't fit us.

David faced Goliath with his familiar sling—and his even more familiar trust in God's abilities. While not a trained soldier, David's love and trust provided the courage to face a giant.

Most of us aren't trained medical professionals—and we don't have to be. When facing our giants, we can be ourselves and, with love and trust, remain confident the battle is the Lord's.

• • •

> *"All those gathered here will know that it is*
> *not by sword or spear that the LORD saves;*
> *for the battle is the LORD's."*
> *—1 Samuel 17:47 NIV*

7

Not Making It Worse Counts as a Win

· · · · ·

As caregivers, we regularly feel intense pressure to fix or achieve. Yet, despite our best efforts, many of the circumstances we face seem unyielding. Our self-judgment over things beyond our control often leads to an incorrect verdict of failure.

Taking a step away from the caregiver realm, consider the "Slap heard around the world" at the 2022 Academy Awards. When Will Smith assaulted Chris Rock on stage in front of a global audience, Chris Rock responded with extraordinary restraint. Maintaining his composure, Chris Rock continued with the show and walked away with nearly universal approval because he didn't worsen an awful situation. Not only did he handle himself well on stage, but in the ensuing media frenzy, he remained quiet about the event. Rock chose to address the incident on his timing—when temperatures cooled.

As caregivers, we regularly face situations that often tempt or provoke us into intense emotional reactions. Taking a page from Chris Rock, we can incorporate a simple strategy with uncontrollable experiences: **Not making it worse counts as a win!**

When we restrain our emotions and master our response to any given circumstances, we live a bit calmer and can add more victories to the "win column."

• • •

Liberty exists in proportion to wholesome restraint. —Daniel Webster

8

A Time for Everything

• • • • •

While checking on my wife during rounds following a significant surgery, the neurosurgeons inquired how things were going. With a serious expression, I inquired if *Tourette's Syndrome* was a complication of this surgery. Gracie hoarsely and indignantly whispered she did not have *Tourette's Syndrome*! Even through their masks, the smiles of the surgical team lit up the room. For a moment, laughter distracted us all from the hardship of her recent surgery—and her considerable pain.

Gracie is keenly aware of the seriousness of her challenges and hardly needs me to remind her. However, she does require a lifeline to brighter days ahead and companionship along the journey. Hence, I tease and flirt outrageously with her—even in a hospital. She weakly smiled and rolled her eyes at me when I imitated Jeff Foxworthy and said, "If you hang a sock on your wife's hospital room door, you might be a redneck!"

I couldn't help but notice as she rolled her eyes that tears didn't fill them.

Humor and optimism remain great weapons against despair. While many challenges and heartaches seem permanent, we can still purpose to live with joy, gratitude, and even laughter.

• • •

A time to weep, and a time to laugh.
—Ecclesiastes 3:4 ESV

9

A Bowl of Soup and a Kind Word

· · · · ·

During a challenging hospital stay for my wife, friends called and asked me to stop by their home. After doing laundry, I swung by their house while returning to the hospital. Smiling at my puzzled look, they directed me to the kitchen table, where a single place-setting awaited.

"Your in-laws are caring for your boys, and the hospital staff is caring for Gracie. Sit, eat, and let us care for you." They promptly served me a steaming bowl of vegetable beef soup, a massive slice of cornbread, and a large glass of tea. As a child of the South, they couldn't have picked a better meal for me.

I tried to make conversation but couldn't find the words. "Just eat and rest," they repeated several times.

After finishing the meal, I got up to head back to the hospital, and they both hugged me. "You have a lot to do, but now do it on a full stomach—knowing that you're loved."

Many express difficulties in knowing how to help a caregiver, but most caregivers agree that it's not complicated. Sometimes it's just a bowl of soup and a kind word.

• • •

The angel of GOD came back, shook him [Elijah] awake again, and said, "Get up and eat some more—you've got a long journey ahead of you." —1 Kings 19:7 MSG

10

Don't Take This on Your Next Vacation

• • • • •

While a change of scenery can ease the heartache and struggles of our lives, it's pointless if we pack our resentments and bitterness for the trip. Despite Yellowstone National Park's pristine and soul-stirring beauty, visitors still bring their drama to the faraway fields of bison and Old Faithful. A sad set of statistics for the world's first national park is the number of drunk drivers and domestic abuse cases handled yearly. Park rangers will undoubtedly affirm that people pack their strife with them—misery's jurisdiction doesn't end at any park's borders.

It's hard to imagine saving up all year long and going to the trouble of traveling so far, only to end up standing in front of one of the federal judges in the park.

While tempted to express disapproval of those arrested for such things in Yellowstone Park, how is that different for many caregivers who think a change of scenery—or circumstances—can serve as an anti-dote for discord?

Yet, if misery can be carried, it can also be put down.

There is no vacation destination that will cure bitterness. The spectacular cannot accomplish what we refuse to implement. We can better appreciate the beauty in different locations once we choose to experience them in our current situation.

• • •

The world is full of people looking for
spectacular happiness while they snub
contentment. — Doug Larson

11

Healthiness in Your Hands

· · · · ·

The neediness of an infirmed loved one frequently obscures a caregiver's fatigue, stress, and dangerous health patterns. Moreover, even if noticing the caregiver's exhaustion and strain, those warning signs often go unheeded. Usually armed only with love and a sense of responsibility, caregivers recklessly deplete themselves physically and emotionally while caring for a vulnerable loved one. Passion and commitment are admirable, but how long can the patient "feel better" at the caregiver's expense?

When faced with chronic impairments, love and responsibility accomplish more when directed to the caregiver's well-being *first*. However, many caregivers postpone healthy physical, emotional, and even sound fiscal decisions for themselves while in the throes of caregiving. Since no one else—particularly a sick or medicated individual—can lead the efforts toward one's own healthiness, the responsibility of a healthy lifestyle remains solely in the caregiver's hands.

Addressing the caregiver's needs (not wants) isn't selfish. Quite the opposite—it helps ensure that the impaired loved one's care is in the hands of a healthier caregiver.

• • •

The first wealth is health.
—Ralph Waldo Emerson

12

A Path Through the Storm

• • • • •

When storms loom, media outlets often show footage of people placing plywood on homes and businesses and hunkering down. Caregiving is its own storm. Although sometimes receiving advance notice, caregiving can often descend like a tornado—and last a lifetime. If cameras followed caregivers, many daily activities might resemble the frantic bustle of those boarding homes and businesses. Imagine trying to build a five-year plan while simultaneously working to survive a hurricane. Incredulously, many caregivers regularly attempt such a feat. While the aftermath of hurricanes usually brings clearer skies that allow rebuilding, the lengthy caregiving storm usually ends at a cemetery—and the path to rebuilding appears shrouded in confusion, despair, and even desolation.

Yet a path through and following the storm does exist. It's called endurance. The challenges of caregiving can forge a resilience and resolve that spills into every area of life. Many faced with hardships lament, "How do I get out of this?" Caregivers (and others) can instead change that question to "What can I become through this?"

Entire marketing ads promote tempting versions of success that sadly ring hollow as the years pass. Endurance remains its own success while standing the test of time.

● ● ●

> *. . . knowing that suffering produces*
> *endurance, and endurance produces*
> *character, and character produces hope . . .*
> —*Romans 5:3–4* ESV

13

Risk Is a Part of Life, but Joy Is a Choice

• • • • •

"Happy New Year" can often feel perfunctory and even meaningless in the caregiving world. Most of us know that January 1, 2, 3, etc., usually brings the same challenges as the previous week and year(s).

Yet although our responsibilities may not change, we can.

While many fall into the trap of ambitious but unrealistic New Year's Resolutions (I usually give mine up for Lent), caregivers can instead determine to live rather than just survive.

Living, however, requires risks. Life is perilous— despite our culture obstinately working to mitigate all risks (thank the lawyers for that). Isolating to avoid disease, injury, rejection, or failure is no way to live. Nor is avoiding death the same as living.

From gardening to music, anything that involves life, art, and creativity comes with the risk of failure, as do relationships, business ventures—and caregiving.

This year, I intend to push myself to learn, try, accomplish—and even fail—new things. History teaches that risks and heartache remain unavoidable, but joy is a choice.

• • •

"It ain't dying I'm talking about, it's living.
I doubt it matters where you die,
but it matters where you live."
—Augustus McCrae, from Lonesome Dove
(Larry McMurtry)

14

The Promise

· · · · ·

Many caregivers struggle with decades-old promises to make sure to "never put Mom in a nursing home." When making that promise, most recall healthier times when the thought of entering a facility seemed far on the horizon. Reality sneaks up on the best of us, and we find ourselves faced with uncomfortable circumstances.

The promise's tether can quickly transform into a noose around the neck of a family caregiver unable to meet the demands of a horrific condition. From personal safety to medical expertise, caregivers easily find themselves outmatched by an affliction—and overpowered by guilt.

Despite the promise's sincerity, its roots often stem from ignorance about the peripheral havoc disease and injury can cause. Disparity and unsustainability quickly appear when a caregiver demands of herself what an entire paid staff of people in a memory care facility accomplish. The promise must face honest scrutiny to reflect the commitment to caring for a loved one to the best one can. When demands exceed ability, changes must occur—and help enlisted.

The challenge for caregivers is seeking counsel from objective, experienced, and trained individuals to regularly evaluate conditions and possible paths.

As we promise to care, let us also commit to caring well.

• • •

We cannot direct the wind, but we can
adjust the sails. —Dolly Parton

15

Not So Silent Night

• • • • •

A reporter once asked me, "What would Jesus do as a caregiver?" Despite the question seemingly arriving from left field during the interview, I responded, "I don't know what He would do, but I can tell you what He *did* do."

Referencing Jesus assigning care of His mother to the apostle John, I said, "He delegated and ensured Mary's care—from the cross."

We think of a pastoral scene for the nativity at Christmas. In reality, the event must have frightened both Joseph and Mary. Most scholars agree that Mary was only a teenager. As a carpenter and not a shepherd, Joseph probably possessed few birthing skills—and the conditions were indeed less than ideal.

During that "not so silent night," Mary trusted the Almighty as she delivered the child who would one day deliver her.

Amid His agony on the cross, Jesus remembered His mother—and her sorrow, pain, and fear. He also enlisted the help of a trusted friend, John, to care for her.

Christmas often comes with sadness for many. Yet there is comfort in knowing that same Savior who saw to His mother's need also sees ours—even when our nights are not so silent (or holy)! We also can discover He has already delegated others around us to help.

● ● ●

Yet in thy dark streets shineth, the everlasting
light. —"O Little Town of Bethlehem,"
Phillips Brooks

16

Thinking on Our Feet

· · · · · ·

A stabbing pain beside my left little toe once prompted a visit to a podiatrist.

"You have a bunion by your left big toe," he stated flatly.

"I know about my bunion; I named it 'Paul,'" I replied, laughing. "But it doesn't hurt. The pain is on the other side of my foot."

"You don't understand," he responded. "The defect of the bunion causes the pain you feel." Patiently explaining, he added, "The bunion affects your walking gait and creates stress points that cause pain. I'll bet your left knee hurts too, doesn't it?"

Admitting it did, I listened while he described treatment plans to help relieve the problem.

Discomfort with the pressures of caregiving often leads many caregivers to blame the loved one—the "pain point." However, with an honest look, we find the culprit is often our predisposition to fear, worry, and control. Those defects disrupt our balance, and are often greatly amplified by the stress of caregiving.

The doctor helped identify and treat the root issues of my foot's pain, and the discomfort eased. With his help, I improved the way I walk.

I also learned that when focusing on the root cause of my stress—invariably my defects instead of others'—I improve the way I live.

● ● ●

Once we know ourselves, we may learn how
to care for ourselves. —Socrates

17

Quieten the Room

· · · · ·

"We've done everything possible to save this leg; all that's left is amputation—when you're ready, we'll have that conversation."

Those words came from Gracie's surgeon, following numerous operations to save her right leg that was crushed and disfigured in her 1983 car accident. Everyone in Gracie's life, including me, had an opinion about this—and Gracie understandably struggled mightily during this time. At twenty-five, with a toddler, the decision weighed heavily on her young heart.

Setting an appointment with our pastor, Bob, she limped into his office on her mangled right foot. As she sat quietly in his study, he stated, "Gracie, this room is off-limits to every other voice telling you what to do. My job is to help quieten the noise so you can hear your heart and God's leading."

Gracie pondered for more than an hour while Pastor Bob sat at his desk—no words passed between them. Finally, Gracie looked up with tear-filled eyes and said, "I'm terrified of doing this," she whispered.

Gaining strength, she continued, "But I can't live this way any longer—it's got to come off."

Nodding somberly, he assured Gracie he'd be with her through the ordeal—and he kept his word.

Sometimes the greatest gift we can give to others struggling with heartbreaking decisions is to clear the room, quieten the noise, and sit with them. Most know what needs to be done but need a quiet place to process the fear and heartache while assured they're not alone.

• • •

Be still, my soul; the Lord is on your side;
bear patiently the cross of grief or pain; leave
to your God to order and provide; in ev'ry
change he faithful will remain. Be still, my
soul; your best, your heav'nly friend through
thorny ways leads to a joyful end.
—"Be Still, My Soul,"
Katharina von Schlegel

18

Assure Rather Than Argue

• • • • •

Do you ever listen to talk radio or cable news when the panel starts to argue? The voices become an unsettling "wall of noise," and most change the channel in seconds. If we're annoyed by talking heads shouting over politics, imagine the unsettledness of those with cognitive issues engaging in or listening to arguments.

When dealing with someone with an impairment, all kinds of subjects fly into the conversation. From seeing things not there to recalling things inaccurately, it remains pointless to argue when cognitive decline is present. Even in the presence of brilliant oratory, the impairment still wins the battle. Rather than pointlessly escalate blood pressure, tensions quickly diffuse when assuring instead of arguing.

Being *right* is a poor substitute for being *there*. Like all of us, people with cognitive issues find themselves unsettled but often cannot process those circumstances or problems. The human condition eventually leads us into places of fear and confusion where we all desperately need assurance—despite our abilities or inabilities. Ironically, we often discover more assurance for ourselves by offering it to others in distress.

• • •

Peace is not absence of conflict; it is the
ability to handle conflict by peaceful means.
—Ronald Reagan

19

Some Days You're the Statue—Other Days You're the Pigeon

• • • • •

It's often repeated, "We demand justice for others but mercy for ourselves." Despite all our technological advances and the heralding of our evolution, the human condition remains fraught with one-sided grievances. Our machines change but our character, sadly, stays the same.

In my journey, I notice the shortcomings of others appear in 20/20 focus, while I apply a much softer filter to my own.

Blaming others for disappointments is easy—and justifiable at times. Yet I learned bitterness does nothing to improve my contentment and well-being. Although it seems counterintuitive, a friend shared an effective way to live peacefully is by concentrating on "cleaning my side of the street."

A tremendous mental shift occurred when I looked hard at my offenses rather than focusing on others. I painfully discovered that while I was the statue some days, other days I regretfully was the pigeon.

Although disappointment remains a constant in this world, grace is optional. We become gracious when extending to others the same grace we desire for ourselves.

• • •

Man is born broken. He lives by mending.
The grace of God is glue. —Eugene O'Neill

20

Your Family May Consider YOU the Solution

· · · · ·

Dear Peter:

> My family lives out of state but complains I am not taking care of my 96-year-old mom, who lives alone by choice. While I help her, she will not authorize a power of attorney for health care. She has no significant medical problems, yet my family is ridiculously harsh toward me and accuses me of things I haven't done or puts pressure on me for things that are not my responsibility. What do you recommend? —Exasperated in Texas

Dear Exasperated:

- Does any agreement about the division of responsibilities exist in your family?
- What exactly is your family accusing you of doing or not doing?

- What type of solutions do they offer?
- Are you aware of efforts on their part to accomplish any tasks (power of attorney, staffing, etc.)?

These seem to be important questions to answer. Until they help provide solutions, it appears your family considers YOU the solution—while also feeling free to criticize you for not fulfilling their expectations.

Before stewing in resentment, it's best to clarify expectations and responsibilities. If you feel uncomfortable doing this yourself, please seek help from an experienced social worker, clergy, attorney, or another objective party.

• • •

The single biggest problem in communication
is the illusion that it has taken place.
—George Bernard Shaw

21

When We Rob Ourselves

· · · · ·

One of the greatest thefts to family caregivers comes from our own hearts. We often steal from the moment to regret the past—or fear the future. Although yesterday's events may have arrived with tears and trauma, today remains an opportunity to calm our hearts and deal with current circumstances. As caregivers, we all know our tomorrows most likely show up with challenges—but unexpected joys may also arrive.

Surprising beauty awaits us along the way, yet we are sure to miss it when our focus extends behind or in front of us. None of this eliminates the grief we carry. However, healthily living in the present allows us to mourn while simultaneously resisting the fear, rage, and despair that often erupts during caregiving.

Although our independence, relationships, career paths, and even dreams inevitably suffer in our caregiving journey, peace of mind remains solidly in our hands. No one has the power to rob us of that composure—except ourselves.

• • •

We know what we are but know not what
we may be. —William Shakespeare

22

Rushing to the Side of an Injured Soul

● ● ● ● ●

Famed anthropologist Margaret Mead shared that "the first sign of civilization is compassion, seen in a healed femur." She backed her claim by explaining the amount of time and compassion required from the tribe or community to care for that individual until able to resume normal activities.

"Survival of the fittest doesn't include healed femurs."

Caregivers live with significant injuries and wounds of the soul that can cripple a person. Anyone who's cared for a chronically impaired loved one cannot recover from such an experience without compassionate help from others. Just as we would rush to someone with a broken leg and respect the time needed for recuperation, caregivers also need others to run to their side.

For caregivers, trauma can extend far beyond a funeral. Although many well-wishers are friendly to caregivers, being nice is a learned behavior—not a sign of character. During and in the aftermath of caregiving, family caregivers need (and deserve) more than "nice." They cry out for compassion and grace—and the recovery may take a while.

Offering compassion and grace helps heal a caregiver while simultaneously deepening the hearts of those extending mercies.

• • •

Teach me to feel another's woe, to hide the fault I see, that mercy I to others show, that mercy show to me. —Alexander Pope

23

Their Happiness Isn't Your Responsibility

• • • • •

Dear Peter:

My 93-year-old mother doesn't suffer from dementia but is so mean to me. How do I make her happy while caring: for her? I've been sober for six years, and she makes me want to start drinking again. —Terri in Texas

Dear Terri:

Your responsibility is not to make your mother happy but to work on your sobriety program. Your mother can get happy in the same shoes she gets mad in! Your responsibility is to call your sponsor and continue staying sober. If you lose sobriety, your mother gets a drunk caregiver, and your circumstances deteriorate further.

The guilt you feel—or your mother wants you to feel—will only drag you into a dark place filled with resentment and despair that you will want to soothe with alcohol. Call your sponsor and go to a meeting.

• • •

Strength of mind rests in sobriety; for this keeps your reason unclouded by passion.
—*Pythagoras*

24

Avoid Living in the Wreckage of Our Future

· · · · ·

Over my wife's thirty-plus years as an amputee, we've learned astonishing things about the human body, including phantom-limb pain. Amputees can often feel the sensations and pain of a limb long since removed.

In what might be described as "reverse phantom limb pain," caregivers often feel anguish over things that haven't even occurred. Caregiving stress is hard enough without us adding to it by living in the wreckage of our future. Letting our imaginations run wild with all sorts of things that may happen wreaks havoc on us and keep us in a constant state of agitation.

Each day often brings circumstances that tempt us to act out of fear and its frequent companion: rage. But we are not doomed to those behaviors. Each day can also offer the opportunity to respond rather than react.

My martial arts instructor often shared in training seminars, "Fight what's closest—not what's beyond our reach." It's a waste of time and resources to focus on battles that don't exist, particularly when plenty of challenges daily stare us in the face.

• • •

"Therefore do not worry about tomorrow,
for tomorrow will worry about itself.
Each day has enough trouble of its own."
—Matthew 6:34 NIV

25

The Adult in the Room

• • • • •

A caller named Bill once shared on our caregiver program that his father was an abusive alcoholic for years. His father has now suffered a stroke and requires extensive care—but sadly still drinks. Even though Bill is over fifty with a wife and kids, he shared that he still feels like a terrified nine-year-old when he's around his father.

Bill's dad made his own decisions—ones that evidently did not involve a recovery plan. I shared with Bill that he can only do his best, but his family needs the fifty-year-old version of BILL—not the nine-year-old one.

Bill's well-being remains paramount to his family. To be blunt, while desirable, his father's well-being does not.

Although it sounds harsh, the reality is Bill's dad may not make it, but Bill must. I commended Bill for ensuring his father's safety and care despite the trauma the man caused. But I also cautioned Bill on the importance of securing his own care and well-being by attending a recovery program for family members of alcoholics and even counseling.

Honoring your mother and father does not mean honoring alcoholism, addiction, or even abuse.

• • •

It's ironic how we can still get hurt by
something we've seen coming. —Anonymous

26

Pushing Back
against the Isolation

• • • • •

Due to Covid-19, the world discovered what caregivers already knew: isolation fosters dark thoughts that easily take us down—often quickly. Pushing back on isolation as a caregiver, however, usually requires creativity. Sometimes it is as simple as a Facebook group, but that can only go so far. Regular phone, face-to-face conversations, and, when possible, group events serve as the path toward healthy engagements.

It's also best to start slow and avoid pinning our hopes on a single individual or encounter. Isolation often makes our hearts feel "parched," and it's tempting to "guzzle" human contact. When dehydrated, it's best to sip water slowly and give our bodies a chance to hydrate appropriately.

The same thing applies to interaction. We serve ourselves (and others) better when resisting the urge to make friends drink from the fire hose and listen to every detail of our journey as a caregiver. Speaking slowly and calmly will ease us into a healthy engagement with others. Isolation remains a constant challenge for caregivers, but one we can regularly defy with something as simple as a telephone.

● ● ●

Walking with a friend in the dark
is better than walking alone in the light.
—Helen Keller

27

Caregiver Advice— Montana Style

• • • • •

During our first winter in Montana, a friend gave me some of the best advice about the snowy road conditions in the Treasure State.

"Drive at the speed you're comfortable slamming into the ditch at."

While laughing at the pointed guidance, I also considered the implications for other areas. As caregivers, we often race around at breakneck speeds— while in treacherous conditions. Relationships, money, and our health can all be severe hazards. The faster we move, the greater the risks.

Slowing down is the key. We make few, if any, sound decisions when we are "amped up." Just like wildlife jumping in front of our trucks, life has a way of hurling things in front of us as caregivers. Slowing down allows us to protect ourselves better, our property, and our loved ones—and the occasional deer in the road! Ditches and wrecks can't always be avoided, but we can reduce the damage.

Besides, going slower allows us to better see the beauty around us.

• • •

Let thy step be slow and steady, that thou stumble not. —*Tokugawa Ieyasu*

28

Advice about Fretting from a Bass Player

• • • • •

A drummer friend from Nashville named Richard recounts the journey to a gig with a bass player named Roy. Repeatedly looking at his watch, Richard fumed about getting to the event hall on time. Meanwhile, Roy just kept driving. Fifteen minutes before they were supposed to arrive, they still had a thirty-minute drive. Growing increasingly anxious, Richard muttered about how late they were.

Bass players are often known to be a bit mellow, and Roy was no different. In a soft Tennessee drawl, Roy quietly said to the frenetic drummer, "We ain't late yet."

Richard had to smile. Recognizing he fretted over something that had not yet happened, he saw how needlessly miserable he made himself (and others). While punctuality and time are undoubtedly important (particularly for drummers), Richard learned a lesson that day about worrying.

As caregivers, how often do we worry about things before they occur? When racing to meet deadlines and timetables, the tendency to fret usually overtakes me. In my better moments, I try to recall those words from Roy: "We ain't late yet."

● ● ●

There were many terrible things in my life
and most of them never happened.
—Michel de Montaigne

29

You Can't Push a Wheel-chair with Clenched Fists

· · · · · ·

There's nothing quite like caring for someone with challenges or impairments to expose the gunk in one's soul. Regardless of our best intentions, when selfishness rears its ugly head, our jaws can quickly tighten—and our fists clench.

As a pianist, my hands must always remain open to make beautiful music. As caregivers, what kind of music do we forfeit when resentment curls our hands into fists?

Try pushing a wheelchair with clenched fists. (Not with your loved one in it—use an empty one!) It's challenging to do so. Clenched fists accomplish few tasks; it seems fighting is the only suitable task for them.

Caregiving will push all our buttons. People who tell you differently haven't done it long enough. Yet, in those moments when seeing our character defects, we can remind ourselves to unclench our fists—and hearts—and allow beautiful music to flow from our souls.

• • •

> *Let it hurt. Let it bleed. Let it heal.*
> *And let it go.* —*Unknown*

30

"To Sell or Not to Sell . . ."

• • • • •

A friend called to discuss her sister in another state who took care of their mother. The mother passed away, and the sister was conflicted about buying out the rest of the family and keeping their house. My friend added, "She doesn't make much money, and it's a large house. What are your thoughts?"

While vigorously avoiding dispensing financial advice (and advice in general), I shared with my friend that I never learned much about real estate while studying music in college. I added, "I have learned (painfully) a lot about the cost of making business decisions based on emotional attachments."

Going further, I offered, "If the house is a solid business venture for your sister, it might make sense for her to finance it, buy you out, and keep it as it grows in value. However, if she does this for emotional reasons, it will most likely be a physical and financial burden to her."

Part of grieving is letting go. For this sister, the healthier path may be to sell it, mourn the loss, and rejoice at the weight she no longer carries.

Emotions and attachments can entangle issues and create long-term hardships that short-term (and healthy) mourning would prevent.

● ● ●

The truth of the matter is that you always know the right thing to do. The hard part is doing it. —Norman Schwarzkopf

31

Don't Pass the Snowplow

· · · · ·

Grabbing my coat to head out into the falling snow following a meeting, I heard a friend call out, "Don't pass the snowplow!

I usually choose a safer road in heavy snow, but my wife's wheelchair had a broken crossbar, and I had to get it to the welder's shop for immediate repairs. It was ready and she needed it.

Approaching a large (and treacherous) hill, I took my friend's advice and drove behind the snowplow that serendipitously appeared. Staying back to avoid rocks, salt, and sand, I moved slowly but securely—even down the steep grade on the hill's other side. I arrived at my destination, retrieved the wheelchair, and returned over the freshly plowed hill.

The journey struck me as an excellent picture for caregivers!

The ones who can help us often move slower than we'd like, and it feels like they're listening to elevator music while we crank up Led Zeppelin. Whether a medical provider, counselor, or financial advisor, the safest place is often behind the professionals doing their job—however slowly we may feel they're moving.

• • •

Patience is the ability to idle your motor
when you feel like stripping your gears.
                    —*Barbara Johnson*

32

When Caregivers Reach the Boiling Point

• • • • •

Every caregiver recalls moments when harsh words flew from our mouths—words we desperately wish to reclaim. Emotions often churn in our hearts like a blender on puree, and, for caregivers, the top seems to fly off and create a mess. Whether expressing frustration or just reaching a boiling point, we can quickly find ourselves spewing words like a firehose—often destructively.

Arguing with an impaired loved one suffering from dementia, mental illness, or addiction is pointless. Unleashing our vexations on family, friends, coworkers, or medical providers only heaps more guilt and sorrow on our already bruised hearts, yet we still need to express ourselves.

The healthier outlet for these feelings is with a trained mental health professional, support group (even a virtual one), clergy, or a trusted friend. We may have to hold our tongues between those safe moments—albeit with great effort. However, the good news is that we rarely need to make amends for something we didn't say.

• • •

> *Speak when you are angry and you will*
> *make the best speech you will ever regret.*
> *—Ambrose Bierce*

33

The Toughest Challenge

• • • • •

A reporter asked me, "What's the toughest challenge you've faced as a caregiver?"

"Knowing what's mine—and not mine—to carry," I replied without hesitation.

Surprised at my answer, he asked for clarification.

"I've spent a lifetime overreaching and trying to carry, fix, and solve things that are not mine," I shared.

Gracie's accident happened before I met her. I didn't do this to her, nor can I undo this. Despite navigating this for nearly forty years, I still haven't even slowed it down—much less solved the problem. Yet fear drove me to recklessly hurl myself toward trying to repair the irreparable. In the process, I made myself miserable and caused great heartache for others—particularly Gracie.

Years ago, I looked down at my hands, noticed no nail prints scarring them, and accepted that this was not mine to fix—it's way above my paygrade. That day, I began seeing myself as a steward, not the owner of this medical nightmare. The choking fear that often gripped me became quelled by the conviction that His scarred hand tightly holds my scared hand.

God alone can alleviate Gracie's challenges. My role is to care for her while trusting His provisions as we wait for Him to do so.

Whether through fear, guilt, or some heightened sense of responsibility, it seems many fellow caregivers push themselves to extremes in vain efforts to wrap their arms around something beyond our abilities to hold.

When the illusion of control tempts me "punch above my weight class," I'm anchored back into reality with words a wise friend once told me: "She has a Savior . . . *you* are not that Savior."

• • •

Never be afraid to trust an unknown future
to a known God. —*Corrie ten Boom*

34

Caregivers and Conflict

• • • • •

In ancient times, numerous civilizations developed a sport where teams pulled on opposite ends of a sturdy rope, and victory went to the team overpowering the other. This activity, commonly referred to as "tug-of-war," exists today. Webster's dictionary describes this activity as "a struggle for supremacy or control usually involving two antagonists."

Not limited to teams with ropes, this "struggle for supremacy" extends into virtually every relationship, including family caregivers—particularly those dealing with cognitive impairment or addiction issues. The war of wills adds increased stress to an already stress-filled environment.

In tug-of-war, winners often land on their rears, and losers often fall flat on their faces. Since the two possible outcomes of landing on one's rear or face present undesirable results, only one alternative exists for family caregivers when faced with a tug-of-war relationship . . .

Don't pick up the rope.

• • •

It is honorable for a man to stop striving,
Since any fool can start a quarrel.
—Proverbs 20:3 NKJV

35

Reality Always Trumps the Hypothetical

· · · · ·

Dear Peter:

"If you could, would you go back and do it all again as a caregiver?? —Chip, feeling reflective

Dear Chip:

As caregivers, we struggle enough with reality, so living in the hypothetical is never recommended. That said, I love how I play the piano now, I love how I write, and I am grateful for how I can speak to fellow caregivers—yet I often hate how I got here.

I'm learning to be grateful for the journey because it brought a texture to my life I wouldn't have without those experiences. I notice and value beauty I would have probably missed, and I see purpose in my journey—the purpose of becoming a better person because of my path as a caregiver.

My questions also changed, and I abandoned asking, "Why?" and "How do I get back to normal?" The recurring question is, "What can I become through this?"

Time and perspective allow me to live more peacefully with the challenges. That peace helps put aside all hypothetical musings.

• • •

Life is not a problem to be solved,
but a reality to be experienced.
—Søren Kierkegaard

36

The Caregiver FOG

• • • • •

Slowing down tops the list of directives from the National Weather Service to drivers encountering fog. Furthermore, they recommend using low beam lights because high beams create a glare.

Caregivers often find themselves in a "fog." While fog consists of water vapor, the "caregiver FOG" consists of fear, obligation, and guilt. Without exception, every caregiver will experience these difficult feelings in their journey. Yet the National Weather Service directive also applies to family caregivers.

When disoriented by the caregiver fog, slow down and try not to see too far ahead. While fear of the unknown twists us in knots, feeling obligated quickly leads to resentment. Furthermore, the amount of guilt torturing caregivers is heartbreaking. These feelings can cause us to career off the road and into danger.

Slowing down while giving ourselves space and grace in dealing with what's directly in front—helps us better navigate the fog of caregivers.

• • •

*Drive slow and enjoy the scenery—drive fast
and join the scenery. —Douglas Horton*

37

Boundaries and Addicts

• • • • •

A listener shared, "We've agreed to let our nephew live with us for a year following his release from prison on drug charges. My husband's had significant health issues, and I could use the help. Although we see real changes in him, we're still nervous. What are your thoughts?"

Thinking about this couple's challenge, I offered, "Enabling—like an addiction—can convince you 'you don't have that problem.' Your nephew may demonstrate real change, but boundaries are your most effective tool in dealing with him."

I explained further, "Working a recovery program, paying for food/rent, and helping with housework/maintenance remain a must for your nephew. In addition, it would be wise to prohibit him from bringing over guests for a predetermined time. The best chance of success is to provide him with a written list of expectations while explaining that those items remain nonnegotiable. His feelings don't get a vote on your boundaries."

Lastly, I referred this couple to a twelve-step program for family members of alcoholics—an excellent resource to attend immediately.

Compassion often causes many hearts to feel conflicted about making tough choices and keeping healthy boundaries.

• • •

For each will have to bear his own load. —
Galatians 6:5 ESV

38

The Loss of Identity

· · · · ·

Asking a friend how he felt, he immediately began sharing his wife's diagnosis. After a few minutes of him recounting her "chart," I stopped him while pointedly saying, "I asked how *you felt*."

That's when the tears and the stammering started. Quietly standing as my friend poured out thick emotions, I again witnessed caregivers' difficult struggles with their own identity. Losing ourselves in someone else's story remains a consistent—and hazardous—trap for family caregivers.

That's why I always ask callers to my radio program for caregivers, "How are you feeling?"

By answering in the first person singular, however poorly, that caregiver makes a fundamental move in reclaiming their identity and voice. Even if we stutter or cry while trying to do so, the first step toward becoming a healthier individual—and caregiver—always begins with "I."

Speaking in their own voice allows caregivers to begin a real conversation.

As caregivers, we can often flawlessly recite our loved one's charts but struggle to admit our fear, fatigue, resentment, or grief. Yet rediscovering our own voice is essential to our healthiness as caregivers.

● ● ●

Listen to others, but don't lose your own voice. —Unknown

39

Immeasurable Cost

• • • • •

A close pastor friend of mine called me after burying his beloved dog. While digging the hole, he wept while angrily reflecting on how much he hated death. The conversation turned to the countless funerals he presided over during his ministry—I played the piano for many of those services. We talked a bit longer about some of the cherished families we ministered to during those funerals and discussed our shared anger at death. Then he said something that's never left me.

"Do you know who hates death more?"

"God hates death," he stated quietly.

Pausing, he added, "He hates it so much that He took it upon Himself to provide a way to defeat death."

When Jesus stood at His friend Lazarus's grave, John 11:38 (NIV) shares that He was "deeply moved." Some translations state that anger welled up in Jesus—anger at death.

Mere weeks after standing at Lazarus's tomb, on what we celebrate as Easter Sunday, Jesus indeed conquered death, but at an immeasurable cost to Himself.

• • •

"Please—Aslan," said Lucy, "can anything
be done to save Edmund?"
"All shall be done," said Aslan. "But it may
be harder than you think." —C. S. Lewis,
The Lion, the Witch, and the Wardrobe

40

Words of Life

• • • • •

It seems an increasing trend for our society to invoke removing anything—or anyone—that makes us uncomfortable. Far beyond the "cancel culture," this inclination extends into the fabric of existence. Whether the unborn, or those facing end-of-life through age, disability, or disease, the pressure remains enormous to consider death as a preferred—even dignified—alternative to enduring challenges.

God's Word, however, strengthens and equips us to endure the unimaginable.

We rejoice with and must care for those choosing life. While mourning for those who do not, may we mourn in such a way that those individuals see Christ's compassion reflected in our tears. In their distress, we can gently speak words of life. Yet not to them alone. Caregivers often pour all our encouragement and support into our loved ones and leave little (if any) for ourselves.

What does it look like to build up our own hearts and souls? For me, I often return to old hymns. Often written by people in great distress, many of those hymns beautifully express the soul's cry while anchoring us in the promises of God.

• • •

Beautiful words, wonderful words,
wonderful words of life. —"Wonderful
Words of Life," Phillip Bliss

41

Don't Believe Everything You Think

* * * * *

Experienced pilots quickly affirm how disoriented one can become while flying. All too many tragedies occur when pilots believe their eyes and senses rather than their instruments. Caregivers can also fall into that trap. The segregation of caregiving affects us physically, emotionally, and mentally. It's not just a case of our minds playing tricks on us; isolation robs us of valuable input that promotes better decision-making. English poet John Milton once stated, "loneliness is the first thing which God's eye nam'd not good."

Before man's temptation and fall, God declared that being alone wasn't good.

Despite the directive in Proverbs 3:5–6 (NKJV), "Trust in the LORD with all your heart, and lean not on our own understanding," we still lean on our understanding! A friend often tells me, "Don't believe everything you think!"

Caregiving is too challenging to do alone. If God looked at His new creation and declared man's "aloneness" to be "not good," how much more do we need each other now. Over the years, I've discovered my mind is a dangerous plan to enter alone—I need help from others to sort through conflict feelings and thoughts.

Following a seasoned pilot's example of depending on instruments, the tower, and even a co-pilot, we, in turn, can lean on Scripture, professionals, and friends to help better orient our thinking.

• • •

It is the province of knowledge to speak, and
it is the privilege of wisdom to listen.
—Oliver Wendell Holmes, Sr.

42

Roll Call

· · · · ·

Without mercy, caregivers tend to judge themselves for blunders on the caregiving journey. For a variety of reasons, we ruthlessly push ourselves to achieve perfection against an impossible challenge. Yet, no matter how hard we try, we repeatedly make mistakes and fall short—and we focus only on the bad news of errors. Worse still, we allow others to criticize and heap blame upon our already demoralized hearts.

Caregivers excel at lopsided judgment; we exclusively focus on one side of the equation. While performance remains essential, being present—not perfect—remains our most important contribution.

Many recall responding with "here" or "present" when teachers called the roll at the beginning of class. I'm confident I'm not alone in racing to class before being marked "tardy." An often-repeated quote is, "90 percent of success is showing up." Affirming that point, teachers present an award for perfect attendance at the end of every school year.

Even if we never received such an award as students, we've earned that award as caregivers.

When tempted to "write" a scathing report on your job performance as a caregiver, first take a roll call and recognize who's in attendance.

Even while acknowledging mistakes, it's appropriate for caregivers to present themselves with an award for perfect attendance. That attendance alone reduces the intolerability of a loved one's anguish.

• • •

The presence of another caring person
doubles the amount of pain a person
can endure. —Philip Yancy

43

Stewardship Instead of Obligation

· · · · ·

"I've got to," "I need to," "I have to," "I must," "I should." Every caregiver, at some point, will make these and other similar statements—and, sadly, all too frequently. The feeling of obligation drives us to push ourselves to dangerous stress levels for our health, finances, and emotional stability.

Despite our best efforts at solutions, we usually come up short—mostly because "fixing" the problem often remains way above our paygrade.

As caregivers, we're not owners of the circumstances our loved ones face; we're stewards. Embracing the concept of stewardship frees us to accept we are doing the best we can with what is within our power and abilities.

Feeling obligated quickly makes us resentful, compromising our ability to live healthy lives and serve as healthy caregivers.

However, adopting an attitude of stewardship helps us breathe easier and treat ourselves with mercy—all of which equips us to be better caregivers.

• • •

All the king's horses and all the king's men,
couldn't put Humpty together again.
—Mother Goose

44

What Every Airline Knows

· · · · ·

While flying Delta Airlines to Atlanta years ago, I discovered flight attendants state the best advice for caregivers:

"In the unlikely event of the loss of cabin pressure, oxygen masks will drop from the ceiling. Securely place your mask on first before helping anyone next to you who may need assistance."

That small directive, what I call the "Delta Doctrine," contains applicable wisdom for so many life circumstances—but probably none as poignant as for those of us serving as caregivers. Compassion and love often mistakenly lead us to hold our breath while trying to help someone else breathe. However, once we make that decision, it is only a matter of time before we find ourselves gasping for air. If we are unable to breathe, how can we help anyone else?

Blacking out from lack of oxygen prohibits us from helping anyone. Put our mask on first—seeing to our own safety is not selfish. It's wisdom.

• • •

It is no use saying, "We are doing our best."
You have got to succeed in doing what is
necessary. —Winston Churchill

45

Sometimes It's Not Personal, It's Business

• • • • •

Dear Peter:

How do I get the doctor(s) to really listen to my concerns? Maybe I should start looking for a new one. —Sherri, feeling dismissed

Dear Sherri:

Since changing doctors often creates more challenges, hammering out a good working relationship is preferred to switching—provided they are suited for the job. For every physician visit, I recommend the three "P's."

Be **polite** but not subservient. Medical providers know the science, but you know your loved one.

Be **prepared** with a list of 3–5 pressing issues or questions. Also, dress appropriately. For example, showing up in "Daisy Dukes" and a "Stones" t-shirt sends the wrong message. Wear attire signaling you take the meeting seriously.

Avoid giving opinions on **pharmaceuticals**. While asking questions remains appropriate, allow the medical staff to observe your loved one without your unsolicited input. Although caregivers often learn the vocabulary (and see all the commercials by drug companies), it's best to leave the pharmaceutical conversations to the trained professionals.

All rules have exceptions, but these three reminders are a handy tool to make each medical visit more successful.

• • •

I went to my doctor, you know my doctor—
Dr. Vinny Boombazz. I said, "Doc, I wake up
in the morning, struggle to the bathroom, look in
the mirror, and feel nauseous. What's the matter
with me?" The doc said, "I don't know, but your
eyesight's perfect!" —Rodney Dangerfield

46

They're Not Doing It to You—They're Just Doing It

• • • • •

Detaching from the poor conduct of an impaired loved one remains one of the toughest challenges for family caregivers. Sometimes the behavioral issues stem from chronic pain, dementia, pharmaceuticals, or fear—maybe they're just having a bad day. Regardless of why they behave in such a manner, we don't have to take it personally—even if it sounds personal.

Our emotional health suffers if our self-worth stays tied to someone else's opinion. You are an extraordinary individual, created in the image of God, and—amazingly—you show up to care for an impaired loved one.

Although a caregiver's loved ones may pop off, criticize, or say hurtful things, it's still important to remember they are impaired on some level. Attaching personal value to a sickness, pharmaceuticals, or addiction makes no sense. In most cases, they're not doing it to you—they're just doing it.

Detaching doesn't mean severing—that's amputation. Caregivers' hearts can disconnect from the impairments of a loved one, but it takes help from mental health professionals, clergy, or trusted friends to reinforce that step.

• • •

"We must learn to regard people less in the light of what they do or omit to do, and more in the light of what they suffer."
—Dietrich Bonhoeffer

47

Letting Go of Guilt

· · · · ·

Following a visit with her mother, a woman listening to my show called to share her feelings. "I'm an only child and took care of my father who passed away recently, and now I care for my mother with Alzheimer's," she haltingly shared.

"I feel guilty if I can't make it to see my mother every day at the center."

"Is she safe?"

"Yes," she replied.

"Is she warm, clean, and well-fed?"

"Yes."

"Does she recognize you?"

"Sometimes," she answered sadly.

"Does she recognize the passing of time?"

"Not really."

"If possible, what would they say to you right now?"

Sniffling, she whispered, "They would tell me they love me, to live my life and be successful."

"You've done all you can to honor both your mother and father . . . and care for them," I responded gently. I further added, "Visiting every day is a self-imposed requirement. You're doing the best you can, and by your own statement—they would approve and release you of your guilt." Let go of the guilt—and while mourning the loss, also bask in the love your family shared.

• • •

Calvin: "There's no problem so awful,
that you can't add some guilt to it
and make it even worse." —Bill Watterson,
The Complete Calvin and Hobbes

48

The Small Things to Tackle the Large Problem

· · · · ·

There's a reason they call it "comfort food," and it's often just a refrigerator or drive-thru away. Caregivers become stressed, weary, and discouraged, and we simply want to feel better. While food can provide temporary comfort, indulging in food for relief ultimately harms us further.

That said, it's pointless to create a caregiver diet plan that none of us will follow—but we can make small changes. Maybe that change is avoiding sodas. Make that change, let it take hold, and watch the results. Then make another change, and so forth.

If we're overweight, we didn't get here overnight—and we won't lose the weight overnight, but we can manage the expectations and move slowly in a healthier direction.

However, we may discover that excess weight isn't just around the waist but in the heart. That's the weight that needs to come off first.

• • •

If you can't fly, then run. If you can't run,
then walk. If you can't walk, then crawl. But
whatever you do, you have to keep moving
forward. —Martin Luther King Jr.

49

Laughter: The Best Medicine

· · · · ·

Wheeling my wife into the hospital's elevator, the numerous occupants stared openly at her. Although Gracie is a beautiful woman, I imagined their gawking and awkward silence resulted from seeing her arm in a sling from surgery that morning—as well as the two metal legs emerging below the hemline of her dress. A double-amputee since the 1990s, she long ago made peace with the stares she receives for wearing her prosthetic legs uncovered.

Yet the stares that day seemed more blatant. Just for a reaction, I loudly lamented with a straight face, "Worst hysterectomy ever!"

The passengers immediately stared at their shoes while Gracie rolled her eyes at me. Married for more than thirty-five years, she's learned to tolerate my goofy humor.

When the doors opened, I couldn't resist one more while wheeling her away. With a parting shot at the gaping passengers, I earnestly shouted over my shoulder, "She put up a fight . . . God love her!"

Gracie laughed all the way to the car.

Making a woman laugh that hard after her 80th surgery is a good day's work for a caregiver.

• • •

Laughter is the closest distance between
two people. —Victor Borge

50

Are They Seen?

• • • • •

Hardly the stereotyped smiling, uniformed women pushing the elderly in the park, family caregivers are an often-overlooked army, orbiting every type of chronic impairment. Trauma, disease (including addiction), disorders, and mental illness—look closely, and you'll see a caregiver. Caregiving affects every demographic (even children) without respect for race, religion, gender, or economy.

And ask caregivers how often they get to visit a park.

Admittedly, it's challenging to know what to say to this unpaid and mostly untrained workforce of 65 million Americans. Caregivers themselves struggle with identifying their own needs, and a loved one's challenges often overshadow the caregiver's struggles. Sadly, not knowing what to say leads to nothing said—which perpetuates the isolation. But just a few words could make a huge difference in engaging the weary heart of a caregiver. Sometimes, it is as simple as saying, "I see you and see the magnitude of what you carry—and I hurt with you."

There's little that words can offer to ease a caregiver's challenges. Yet, being seen, appreciated, and respected by others does wonders to bolster the weary heart of caregivers.

• • •

Can I see another's woe, and not be in
sorrow too? —William Blake

51

A Timely Word

•　•　•　•　•

Calls to the authorities tend to be cries for help to control the dysfunctional behavior of a loved one with an addiction or mental illness. Yet the behavior of that individual's caregiver can also be dysfunctional—usually due to the "Caregiver FOG" (Fear, Obligation, and Guilt). Easily losing themselves in this fog (as well as their loved one's chaos), caregivers can quickly become enablers.

Yet, two sentences in the aftermath of a chaotic scene where law enforcement is called might serve as a lifeline to that hand-wringing family caregiver.

"This seems to be taking a real toll on you. Please consider getting counseling and help for yourself—regardless of what happens with your loved one."

While acknowledging the demands on police officers, this suggestion costs nothing, takes only moments, and won't interfere with controlling the scene. A law enforcement officer—an authority figure—can point distraught family caregivers to safety with two mere sentences. In doing so, they quite possibly facilitate a healthier ally in addressing the growing numbers of impaired members of our society.

• • •

If you can't feed 100 people, then feed just one. —Mother Teresa

52

What Will They Think?

• • • • •

How often have we, as caregivers, second-guessed our decisions based on what others may think? While vacillating usually has roots in our insecurities, opinions from others can also contribute to our anxiety. Sometimes, we even torture ourselves with how an impaired loved one will (or would) judge us.

Far from the wisdom of seeking wise counsel, fretting over the opinions of others is an unproductive path that leads to misery. Public opinion can be a cruel taskmaster.

A good rule of thumb for caregivers is to assign value to someone's opinion in equal proportion to the amount of help they provide. Caregivers certainly benefit from the insights of health professionals, clergy, and other trusted sources. Still, a good practice is to weigh "drive-by" caregiving opinions against the source and amount of assistance offered.

Our loved ones and ourselves benefit when we make informed decisions rather than adjust course due to fear of what others may think—what others think is none of our business.

• • •

One man with conviction will overwhelm
a hundred who have only opinions.
—Winston Churchill

53

"But I Didn't Do Anything"

* * * * *

Several years ago, as my wife recovered from one of her surgeries, I chose to sit quietly next to her rather than talking on my phone, working, or doing other frenetic activities that often define me during frequent crisis moments.

Glancing at her, I noticed her breathing stopped, and her face turned blue. Immediately summoning the nurse, who quickly called the code, a flurry of medical staff descended upon the room.

Standing in the corner, I observed a room full of highly trained strangers doing what they do best. As the team stabilized my wife and wheeled her to the ICU, familiar medical staff congratulated me for staying calm and for a job well done.

"You saved her life," they all echoed.

Alone with my thoughts later, I reflected that I didn't do anything—I simply sat there. Yet, my wife is alive because I stopped finding things to keep me busy.

That day, I learned a vital caregiver lesson about the value of being still.

• • •

Never doubt the power of inactivity.
      —*Anonymous*

54

Something Better Than Counting Sheep

● ● ● ● ●

Every caregiver eventually experiences nights where sleep seems elusive. Regardless of fatigue, our racing minds seem reluctant to shut down—and the agitation increases. While fear and anxiety are the main culprits, rage and resentment also lurk nearby. Our weariness, irritability, and even depression seem exponentially greater when morning finally arrives, and we're left to face another day while operating on a deficit of sleep.

Following a particularly long night where I held lengthy conversations with the ceiling fan, a friend gave me some advice.

"Using the alphabet, think of something you're thankful for—that corresponds with that letter."

He added, "Q, X, and Z may give you some trouble, but keep at it—and repeat the process until you drift off."

Although thinking it was a bit too simplistic, I agreed to try. Astonishingly, it worked every time. Furthermore, the simple technique had a spillover effect on my waking hours, and I soon discovered a timeless truth: it's hard to be miserable when you're grateful.

• • •

Gratitude is not only greatest of virtues,
but the parent of all the others.
—Marcus Tullius Cicero

55

Sorry Seems to Be the Flimsiest Word

• • • • •

It appears every news cycle carries another "apology tour" from a celebrity or politician. While many of these *mea culpa*'s make headlines, how many sound sincere?

"I'm sorry if I offended . . ." implies the action isn't considered offensive. Scripted statements like these offer wiggle room for the offender to avoid responsibility. We've all seen it, and I remain unclear why those public spins continue largely unchallenged.

Each of us carelessly blunders. Other times, we intentionally say and do hurtful or even destructive things that cause deep wounds. As caregivers, despite self-sacrifice and noble intentions, we are not exempt from creating carnage in our relationships.

Owning our mistakes and respecting the wounds they cause, while painful, allows us to make sincere amends and grow as individuals. Even while cringing (sometimes for a lifetime), we can focus less on our embarrassment and more on the damage we'd like to repair (if possible).

That's what love does.

Avoiding the "I'm sorry if . . ." and instead stating "I was wrong, and I'd like to make amends" can launch a path toward reconciliation and healing.

• • •

A stiff apology is a second insult—
the injured party does not want to be
compensated because he has been wronged;
he wants to be healed because he has
been hurt. —G. K. Chesterton

56

Patriots Standing
in the Gap

· · · · ·

A recent caller to my radio program shared her journey caring for several grandchildren. Combat-related PTSD led her military son down some dark paths—including drugs and alcohol, and his family disintegrated. This grandmother found herself with both an impaired son and vulnerable grandchildren.

When considering the word "caregiver," most think of caring for the elderly. Yet many kinds of caregivers exist—and each of them bears their own sadness and difficulties.

Throughout the history of militaries, it has been said that soldiers leave a part of themselves on the battlefield. Returning home from the conflict, many struggle to regain normalcy—particularly when dealing with devastating injuries. Sometimes, caregivers push themselves to compensate for the seen and unseen wounds of injured servicemen and women. While our military is composed of volunteers who don the uniform, an additional and less visible army of volunteers exists. Those volunteers are family caregivers who stand in the gap for wounded warriors and their families.

Their acts of devotion serve their loved ones and honor this great nation.

• • •

*There is much more to being a patriot
and citizen than reciting the pledge
or raising a flag. —Jesse Ventura*

57

Are You Paddling Upstream?

• • • • •

Imagine watching someone paddle upstream against a rushing river. The scene might cause us to shake our heads in concern over a person's mental stability trying such a thing.

Yet many family caregivers attempt a similar task while fighting the unstoppable (and often raging) current of Alzheimer's, autism, addiction, or a host of other chronic impairments.

Far from paddling on a lake, caregiving often seems like riding class-five rapids. Before embarking on any white-water trip, good river guides give instructions about not panicking, wearing the proper attire, and moving quickly to keep the raft from flipping when approaching obstacles.

Those same guides will also tell you to enjoy the ride and the scenery along the way.

As caregivers of loved ones with chronic impairments, we can either exhaust ourselves fighting the current—or better position ourselves to move with the water. Caregiving is a bumpy ride. We might as well settle in, wear comfortable clothes, and go with the flow.

And (to our astonishment at times), we can even discover beauty along the way.

• • •

*Don't underestimate the value of doing
nothing, of just going along, listening to all
the things you can't hear, and not bothering.*
—A. A. Milne

58

Playing for Chickens

· · · · ·

There's an old story of a farmer who struggled to find ways to help his chickens lay more eggs. After trying numerous techniques, he heard of the beneficial effects of music and tried playing the flute for his chickens to help them lay more eggs. Sitting beside the coop, he diligently spent hours at a time performing beautiful songs in hopes of providing a better "egg-laying" environment.

After doing this for several weeks, he noticed the number of eggs never changed. Although tempted to be discouraged, he continued playing for his chickens. After watching this activity for some time, a neighbor finally asked the farmer why he kept playing his flute for the chickens when it did not affect their laying eggs.

The farmer replied, "The egg count didn't improve, but my music did."

As caregivers, we may try all sorts of things to improve or help our loved ones. Their challenges, however, remain beyond our control. We can, however, improve ourselves in the journey and quite possibly discover beautiful music along the way.

• • •

When we are no longer able to change
a situation—we are challenged to change
ourselves. —Victor Frankl

59

Hurry Up and Relax

· · · · ·

During the July 4th weekend, one could not help but see the pace quicken as vast numbers of people converged in Montana for vacations. Long lines of campers and trailers left dust plumes while heading into forests to "get away," and traffic horror stories spread from tourist locales such as Yellowstone National Park.

Non-local vehicles fleeing restrictive locales might as well have sported bumper stickers stating, "We need to hurry up and relax!"

As family caregivers, we understand claustrophobic feelings fueled by isolation. The first whiff of fresh air often causes us to bolt toward escapism like horses rushing to the barn following a long ride.

The challenge for caregivers remains the same for pandemic-weary tourists: slow down. Unlike Disney World, for example, Montana's and Wyoming's great gift to the world is the invitation to bask in beauty without frenetic activity. Slowing down, we learn the chaos in our hearts belongs to us—not our loved ones or even the pandemic.

Reducing the pace allows us to discover (and savor) beauty all around us. We can then share that beauty with other weary hearts—and even export it to those unable to travel.

• • •

The most successful people are those who do all year long what they would otherwise do on their summer vacation. —Mark Twain

60

When It's Beyond
My Control

· · · · ·

Two different caregivers shared the same sentiment with me this past week. "I'll get help when it's beyond my control."

When I quietly asked what shape they (and their loved ones) would be at that point, they both gave the same response: silence.

Many caregivers competently (and admirably) handle enormous challenges. The issue, however, is not how competent the caregiver is today. Caregiving takes a considerable toll on physical, emotional, fiscal, and spiritual health. The time to ask for help is not when we're overwhelmed but to seek it in stages long before the critical point.

If my nearly forty years of caregiving has taught me one clear lesson, it's that I needed help from day one. While full-time care isn't always the solution, phasing in care, seeking counsel, or attending support groups are encouraged from the onset of caregiving.

In addition, regular conversations with accountants, one's physician, and clergy are also critical to the caregiver's well-being.

Waiting to seek help until it's "beyond our control" is an illusion.

It was never within our control.

• • •

The way of a fool is right in his own eyes,
but a wise man listens to advice.
—Proverbs 12:15 ESV

61

When It's Hard to See Because of the Forest and the Trees

• • • • •

Following a small job of recently repairing a fence on the ranch in Montana with my father-in-law, I paused for a moment and studied the thick clusters of trees and bushes following a nearby stream. It seemed the trees and bushes all clamored for water in the dry climate of Montana. From my vantage point, I observed the growth stopped about ten yards on either side of the water. Yet, if someone exclusively followed the stream, they might feel claustrophobic or even lost in the thickets—despite being only a stone's throw from clear fields on either side.

Many caregivers find themselves feeling closed in and even lost. While trusted friends, physicians, clergy, or counselors can call to us in those suffocating places, only we can make the leap of faith and move in a new direction. With courage and trust in voices other than our own, we can take steps toward a better perspective that provides clarity and calmness.

That perspective helps us avoid becoming disoriented—even in the dense thickets of caregiving.

• • •

Perspective is everything when you are
experiencing the challenges of life.
—Joni Eareckson Tada

62

Respond Rather Than Anticipate

• • • • •

Trying to predict the behaviors or words of others can often launch us into action before events unfold. A martial arts sparring match once drove this point home for me—somewhat painfully. Feeling certain my opponent would throw a punch, I fixated on his shoulder while mentally preparing my move. To my surprise and embarrassment, he nailed me with a roundhouse kick to the chest.

The discomfort felt on the mat pales to my cringe-worthy events over the same type of behavior as a caregiver. I've lost count of how many times I jumped the gun to quell something before it started, only to get it wrong—and sadly, worsen the situation. Waiting to see how events unfold allows time to respond rather than anticipate a possible outcome and get it wrong. Mistakes on the mat are insignificant compared to hasty judgment as a caregiver.

While action and planning remain essential, we better serve ourselves (and our loved ones) by cultivating the discretion of knowing when to act, speak, or be still.

• • •

What we anticipate seldom occurs;
what we least expected generally happens.
—Benjamin Disraeli

63

Unexpected Leadership

· · · · ·

Following my wife's first amputation thirty years ago, I observed her struggling with inactivity while in the hospital. Despite the challenging injuries leading to the eventual loss of both legs, Gracie consistently demonstrated an action-driven life of accomplishment. As the anxiety and drama leading up to the surgery dissipated, Gracie floundered while considering her plight—yet her surgeon of many years hardly visited.

Until that week, I looked at physicians (particularly surgeons) as quasi-deities. Many of them helped reinforce that belief. But Gracie's struggles prompted an act of unknown courage to confront her surgeon.

"You've been a mainstay in Gracie's life since her accident, and she needs direction right now. If you're not that person, please tell me, and I will find someone else."

Nodding quietly, he added. "I can do that."

Entering her room, he pulled up a chair and spent about an hour with her. I stayed away—that was their time. Afterward, I saw clarity and purpose in Gracie that launched her recovery.

Caregivers often need to provide leadership to those with significant training and authority beyond ours.

• • •

Sometimes, the leader is the one who
remembers where the Jeep is parked.
—US Army saying

64

Serving as a Punching Bag Is Not "Honoring"

· · · · ·

Dear Peter:

The Bible tells us to honor our mother and father, but my alcoholic (and now disabled) father was physically abusive and is still verbally abusive. —David in TX

Dear David:

While one of the Ten Commandments is to indeed honor your father and mother, it does not mean we must honor alcoholism, addiction, or any other type of mental impairment that leads to inappropriate acts. Sometimes honoring them means not engaging in their destructive behavior.

You are not honoring your father by serving as a physical or verbal punching bag, and it's imperative to keep those emotional and sometimes physical boundaries in place. If such an impairment consumes the person, you are not obligated to have a relationship with the disease. Detaching from such a person may lead you to "caregiving from a distance."

In some cases, you may have to honor the person they were—as you care for what they've become.

Regardless of circumstances, "honoring your mother and father" does not license them to abuse you.

• • •

To dispute with a drunkard is to debate with an empty house. —Publilius Syrus

65

Can They or Won't They?

• • • • •

"If only my mother would . . ."

Substitute the word "mother" with father, child, spouse, etc. That phrase rises to one of the most common laments uttered by family caregivers around the globe.

Is the undesired behavior intentional?

Caregivers admit that determining if a loved one "can't do something" and "won't do something" often remains a gray area.

How gray is that area? Charcoal gray.

Regardless, "can't or won't" still leaves caregivers with the challenge of accepting reality versus what we desire. Recognizing the powerlessness to change an impairment or a willful behavior remains a bitter pill for caregivers to swallow.

Although counter-intuitive, the path through this frustration comes not from achieving a desired change in our loved ones but rather a change in ourselves. When our peace of mind remains attached to someone else's actions, we become hostages to their conduct. Yet our freedom remains exclusively in our own hands—and hearts.

Even if their poor behavior results in unpleasant consequences for our loved ones (and sometimes us), we are not required to be miserable while caring for them.

• • •

I don't look for bliss, just contentment.
—Alison Krauss

66

The Weight of Forgiveness

• • • • •

Words matter. All too often, however, words get bandied about with great sentiment but little thought. Of all the weighty words in our vocabulary, *forgiveness* seems one of the least respected. Victims of horrific crimes interviewed during a trial often weep while expressing forgiveness to the perpetrator. Many wounded parties feel pressure from others to "forgive and forget," while others struggle with forgiving themselves.

What does forgiveness even mean?

Forgiveness has weight to it, as well as intentionality. Forgiveness indicates respect for the offense/trauma while being willing to "take your hands off someone else's throat." Forgiveness requires accepting that an offender will receive justice from someone other than yourself—life consequences, the authorities, or God.

Forgiveness benefits the offended, does not require reconciliation, and can be extended even if unsolicited. Remorseless criminals fill our prisons, yet victims can still forgive. Many care for abusive but impaired loved ones who are incapable of repenting and reconciling. Yet those caregivers can still forgive.

Resentment gnaws at our souls. As caregivers, we already bear enough. We can choose instead to walk in forgiveness and lose the grudges—while keeping healthy boundaries.

• • •

To be a Christian means to forgive the
inexcusable because God has forgiven the
inexcusable in you. —C. S. Lewis

67

Major Patience for Major Medical Companies

• • • • •

Dear Peter:

Where does one find the patience to deal with insurance companies? —Myra, feeling claimless in Seattle.

Dear Myra:

Insurance companies are not that complicated. They're businesses driven by financial decisions, not emotional ones. In the throes of caregiving, our emotions run high and often unchecked. When getting on the phone with an insurance representative, remember they have a job to do. You may not like it, and they may indeed be calloused, cold, or seem uncaring. But you don't need them to emote with you; you need them to help facilitate payment of a service, drug, or equipment.

If you must appeal, demonstrate the appeal is in their best financial interest. Every appeal I've won was because it made economic sense for the insurance company. Mostly because approving the appeal kept my wife out of the hospital.

Also, many insurance companies offer a service that assigns a case manager (usually a nurse) to patients with lengthy and extensive medical needs. Ask for such a manager; they will become a great ally to you and your loved one.

● ● ●

The most difficult thing in any negotiation,
almost, is making sure that you strip it
of the emotion and deal with the facts.
—Howard Baker

68

Putting Treasure into a Broken Machine

• • • • •

While attending a weekly support group, I often purchased a soda from a nearby machine. All went swimmingly until one evening when the device failed to dispense the beverage. Disappointed, I called the service number and then joined the meeting. Despite not hearing from the machine's owner, I tried again at the following week's meeting. To my surprise, two soda cans rolled out. Giving one to a friend, I accepted that I "broke even."

I again put coins in the slot a week later—but nothing happened. Exasperated, I "fussed" at and even shook the machine, but to no avail. The following week, I tried once more, but the machine prevailed. I quit putting money into the machine and instead brought a water bottle.

Those with impairments often can't act as they used to or desired. Expecting them to do so sets us up for disappointments and resentments. Coercing, yelling, or swearing remains futile. Yet we continue placing our treasure (self-worth, hearts) into these broken vessels.

Accepting the impairment and making a healthier choice for ourselves is the better path toward peace and contentment.

• • •

Sometimes, expectations can be embryonic resentments. —Anonymous

69

Resistance Is Inevitable

• • • • •

While boundaries remain critical to healthy relationships, they sometimes develop through inaccurate information or impaired thinking. Caregivers inevitably collide with such boundaries while caring for loved ones. These flawed boundaries may look like resisting rehab for injuries or addiction issues, refusing medications, respecting others' time, or a whole host of other issues.

Confronting those disputes requires caregivers' deftness and wisdom, mainly when a loved one is "dug in" behind years of stubbornness. Sometimes, all that's needed is clearly explaining the consequences of behaviors. But when confronting someone with addiction or impairment issues, for example, all many caregivers can do is provide buffers to minimize the damage—while remaining at safe distances as circumstances deteriorate. In other cases, a caregiver must often bite her tongue and learn to like the taste of blood as a loved one experiences the outcome of stubbornness.

Trying to force a solution against someone's will or boundaries usually creates conflict and failure. Despite resistance or even desired results, we can learn to be at peace with our powerlessness over others' boundaries—and instead focus on maintaining our own.

• • •

My happiness grows in direct proportion to my acceptance, and in inverse proportion to my expectations. —Michael J. Fox

70

And the Critics Say . . .

●　●　●　●　●

A friend shared the recent criticism while struggling to care for her husband. Already reeling from significant heartache resulting from her husband's condition, the scolding rocked her.

"You should've done _____."

All too many spectators feel emboldened to offer "advice" to caregivers shouldering the challenges of caregiving. Sometimes non-caregivers bypass advice and go straight to criticizing. I suppose it saves time.

As a rule, the best opinions to heed usually come from those possessing training and education relating to the impairment of your loved one. Almost forty years as a caregiver has taught me an additional rule: the best counsel regarding your journey as a caregiver often comes from those with credible experience.

There remains no shortage of opinions from those not doing the work. Those criticisms, if allowed, can wound the soul of a caregiver struggling to do her best.

When tempted to let critics assess your value as a caregiver by job performance, be fair and look at your attendance record. You keep showing up to care. Critics only show up to judge.

● ● ●

The credit belongs to the man who is actually in the arena, whose face is marred by dust and sweat and blood; who strives valiantly; who errs, who comes short again and again, because there is no effort without error and shortcoming; but who does actually strive to do the deeds. —Theodore Roosevelt

71

Caregiver Authority

• • • • •

Weary of condescension from a physician years ago regarding my wife's condition, I leveled my gaze at him and stated, "With all due respect, Doc—I was taking care of her when you were in junior high school. So how about we keep this in perspective?"

We may not know the science, but we know our loved ones. That knowledge and experience provide us with something I coined "Caregiver Authority." Quality practitioners recognize the benefit of enlisting our hard-won insights. After dealing with 100+ physicians and countless nurses, I learned years ago that training doesn't make one a better human being—it simply provides a skill set. Sadly (for some), those skill sets can elevate a sense of importance. Part of our job as caregivers is to advocate. And sometimes that means standing up to people who are dismissive or look down upon others.

It's uncomfortable to wield caregiver authority, but if we don't, what happens? If we're wrong, we apologize and make amends to the best of our abilities. If they're wrong, the consequences are far more dire.

• • •

> *"I spend half my time comforting the afflicted, and the other half afflicting the comfortable."* —Wess Stafford

72

You Might Be
a Caregiver If . . .

. . . . .

Years ago, while interviewed for AARP, the reporter asked me, "What do you say to those family members who don't realize they are caregivers?"

The question struck me as funny, so I lapsed into my best Jeff Foxworthy impression, "If you have a professional carpet cleaner on retainer, you might be a caregiver!"

Laughing, the reporter said, 'You should do a bunch of those with Jeff."

Longtime friends, I called Jeff and asked what he thought.

"Sure, write some jokes, and we'll do it."

"Jeff, these aren't jokes," I laughed. "This is my life!"

The "You Might Be a Caregiver" we did for AARP was a great success. Here are a few highlights.

- "If you've ever hooked up your wife's wheelchair to your dog—just to see if it would work—you might be a caregiver." (I've done this.)
- "If a hospital bed has never hampered your love life, you're probably a caregiver!' (I plead the fifth.)
- "If at the grocery store, YOU'RE the one asking for a price check on suppositories, you might be a caregiver." (Like you wouldn't!)

On a GOOD day, caregiving can be challenging. Keeping a sense of humor remains critical to staying healthy—and "healthy caregivers make better caregivers."

• • •

If anyone's ever seriously asked you,
"Baby, have you seen my left leg?" . . .
—Jeff Foxworthy

73

Identity Theft and Family Caregivers

• • • • •

According to numerous credit companies, identity theft remains a major headache for individuals and businesses. With America's vast and aging baby-boomer population, the issue of identity theft weighs heavy on seniors—and their caregivers. Individuals and family members show great wisdom when subscribing to various products and safeguards against data breaches.

Yet an overlooked "identity theft" exists for family caregivers. Virtually all caregivers find themselves struggling to speak in their own voice. Ask any family caregiver about how they feel, and one can expect to hear replies using "we," "our," "he," "she," and "us." Using the first person singular of "I" remains one of the most significant challenges for caregivers. Due to various reasons, our own identity can quickly become lost in someone else's story.

On my radio program, we discuss caregivers more than caregiving. I ask every caller, "How do you feel?" Once caregivers learn to speak in their voice, a real conversation can occur and the path to healthiness begins.

Identity theft isn't limited to finances. For family caregivers, it often involves the heart.

• • •

Be yourself—everyone else is taken.
—Oscar Wilde

74

We Can't Change the People Around Us, But . . .

• • • • •

Entrepreneur Jim Rohn once asserted, "You are the average of the five people you spend the most time with." Another famous quote states,

- If you hang around five confident people, you will be the sixth.
- If you hang around five intelligent people, you will be the sixth.
- If you hang around five idiots, you will be the . . .

As caregivers, we owe it to ourselves to inventory the voices with access to our hearts. Although caregivers often find themselves in painful circumstances or surrounded by criticism or other negative attitudes, we can change that.

Recently talking with a man struggling while watching his wife slip away, I said, "You live in an environment permeated by approaching death. Balance that by immersing yourself into life."

Knowing he has great-granddaughters close by, I suggested letting the attendants briefly look after his wife so he can spend time with those precious girls. "The life bubbling out of your great-grandchildren provides a counterweight to your sorrow."

We can't change the people around us, but we can CHANGE the people around us.

● ● ●

Don't walk away from negative people. Run!
—Mark Twain

75

What's Your Melody?

· · · · ·

After my wife stopped singing publicly due to health reasons, our pastor asked me to play the piano before services to help foster a more reverent atmosphere. Sitting at the piano, I launched into a well-known hymn only to quickly discover I wasn't playing the melody.

Accompanying Gracie for years, I'd simply grown accustomed to hearing her sing the melody.

Glancing sideways at the Nashville church filling with hundreds of people, I forced myself to play the melodies of songs I'd known for a lifetime. Yet, the muscle memory in my hands kept reverting to the accompaniment. That ten-minute prelude cost me more musical stress than I'd experienced in years.

Accustomed to "accompanying," caregivers often lose the melody and fail to speak in the first person singular. Like playing the piano, it takes practice—but we can learn to express our own feelings instead of directing every topic to our loved ones. We can learn to speak from our hearts and play our own melody.

● ● ●

You may not control all the events that happen to you, but you can decide not to be reduced by them. —Maya Angelou

76

And the Award for Discretionary Valor Goes To . . .

• • • • •

In trauma, the clock is the adversary, but in caregiving, it's the calendar. While emergencies demand an immediate response, quick actions for caregivers often result in several battles on multiple fronts. Nothing stretches a caregiver too thin like rushing to a crisis while already embroiled in one.

> "Oh, yes, my friend, you would have fought very bravely and died very quickly." —Don Diego to Alejandro in *The Mask of Zorro*

In the long journey of caregiving, caregivers benefit from incorporating "discretionary valor." For many caregivers (including me), the default is to hurl ourselves or our opinions recklessly at situations that require neither. Being still often takes enormous discipline and is its own form of bravery. Although some may not recognize it, knowing when to—or when not to—act often reflects extraordinary wisdom and courage. It's hard to "stay at one's post" when everything is falling apart. Yet one's mettle is usually tested by not interfering when things get dicey. Sometimes, others need to experience failure to grow. Hampering that experience inhibits their growth.

Although not often valued, discretionary valor remains one of the most critical attributes a caregiver can utilize. While soldiers receive medals reflecting bravery under duress, our medals for discretionary valor appear differently. Our awards signify peace of mind, less drama, and a good night's sleep.

● ● ●

Don't just do something; stand there!
—Unknown

77

The Long Valley

• • • • •

Dark thoughts often grip us as caregivers when strug-gling with loneliness and isolation. We fearfully plead for someone to tell us what to do, where to go, how to cope, or why this is happening. Our oldest son fell and lacerated his chin when he was just a tod-dler, and I held him still while he received stitches. I'll never forget the terror in his eyes and his screams as he endured what was horrifying for him. He had no way of understanding what was happening or how to cope. Instead of explaining infections, antibiotics, and wound care, I gently assured him that I was there and he would be okay. Soon, the doctor finished, and I hugged our son and dried his tears.

How are we any different when traveling in the often-long valley of the shadow of death that we walk as caregivers? Our heavenly Father often doesn't give us the answers we demand, but He does give us the assurance we need—the assurance of His presence and love for us.

• • •

Yea, though I walk through the valley of the shadow of death, I will fear no evil: for thou art with me. —Psalm 23:4 *KJV*

78

Acceptance Doesn't Mean Agreement

· · · · ·

Much of the heartache I've endured as a caregiver results from my unwillingness to accept things as they are. Fighting to change things I am powerless to change has only made it harder for me—and, sadly, others.

A friend once told me that acceptance doesn't mean agreement. I may not like what I carry or witness, but I can accept that it is what it is—and be calmer while enduring it. That's not defeatist, just realistic.

My wife helped teach me this when she lost both of her legs. She didn't like being a double amputee, but it became her new reality. Watching her process significant loss and the new challenges, I witnessed her make peace with painful circumstances. While she periodically experiences moments of grief—even decades later—her resolve and acceptance help dry the occasional tears.

As caregivers, acceptance connects our brains to our hearts and allows "what is" to mingle with grief. In the process, we can live more peacefully with the often-chaotic events in our lives—and our resolve to do so can also help dry the more than occasional tears.

• • •

Tears come from the heart and not from the brain. —Leonardo da Vinci

79

We've Got This!

· · · · ·

The morning of the most extensive surgery my wife has ever faced, we both felt (understandably) a bit nervous. Sitting in the pre-op area, I observed a flurry of medical staff work efficiently to prepare Gracie for a nine-hour surgery—and her 82nd operation.

When the neurosurgeon arrived, I noticed a tangible enthusiasm about him. Clapping his hands together, he brightly looked at us while stating, "You ready to get this thing done!"

For maybe the first time in my decades as a caregiver, I felt a calmness and sense of safety with this man. As the surgeon exuded such self-confidence, our anxiety seemed to dissipate. He knew his job and shared his excitement, "I love doing this procedure—it helps so many people!"

Looking at me, he said, 'This will be a long day. Go rest in your hotel room and wait for my call. You don't need to hang out in the waiting room and stress yourself out. We've got this!"

Following his orders, I rested, watched a movie, and waited for his call without worrying about reprisal or condemnation from "pearl clutching" bystanders—a far cry from the harsh judgment I received following my first surgery with Gracie.

The surgery went well, and while slow, the recovery remains steady. Along the way, I learned to trust a bit more—and rest in the competence of others.

• • •

You must trust and believe in people, or life becomes impossible. —Anton Chekov

80

What Do You Think?

· · · · ·

While I've often (and embarrassingly) inserted my opinion during my wife's long medical journey, I don't recall being frequently asked for it—particularly by surgeons. Yet, as the team observed Gracie's responses during the recovery process of her recent surgery, the lead surgeon looked at me and said, "What do you think?"

As her husband and caregiver for nearly forty years, I understand nuances about my wife that no medical professional could hope to know. That said, a lengthy list of unpleasant events continues to teach me the value of keeping my opinion to myself and only sharing what I've witnessed and experienced. So when this surgeon graciously sought my thoughts, I stayed on message, shared what I've observed of my wife and her challenges, and avoided speculating.

Nodding with understanding, he ordered a few additional tests—evidently in part based upon my response—and continued looking for solutions.

As a caregiver, I'm learning to stay in my lane while speaking with calm authority about what I know—recognizing my experience is worth far more than my opinion.

• • •

We have no right to express an opinion until
we know all of the answers. —Kurt Cobain

81

Stillness or Illness

* * * * *

Years ago, my father pastored in Atlanta, and I still recall the oppressive and sweltering Georgia summers. Oscillating fans mounted high on the church walls gently buzzed throughout his sermons, and I'm sure he sighed while looking down and seeing all five of his sons sacked out to the world during his sermons. To this day, a fan puts me to sleep quicker than even Nyquil. I'm not alone in this—electronic devices such as Amazon's Alexa can play fan noises.

With clamor around us, isn't it odd that the gentle sound of fans can lull us to sleep and promote calmness? Television, music, sirens, phones, construction, and traffic form a wall of sound that creates agitation.

Noise pollution only adds to the anxiety and sensory overload we experience as caregivers, which can eventually make us sick. Ask any healthcare professional about the long-term effects of stress. Does anyone tout the benefits of anxiety, high blood pressure, depression, skin rashes, or other stress-induced issues?

As caregivers, if we don't take time for stillness, we will have to make time for illness. Yet being still and quiet requires intent and discipline. The benefit, however, is that it helps re-boot our minds and hearts. Without any cost or even a prescription, regularly incorporating stillness calms us down and equips us to live healthier.

Also, box fans are much cheaper than medication and doctor visits.

● ● ●

The best cure for the body is a quiet mind.
—Napoleon Bonaparte

82

When the Phone Feels Like 100 Pounds

• • • • •

Despite living in dire need of assistance, many caregivers struggle with asking for—and receiving help. Six core reasons serve as stumbling blocks for caregivers when asking for help, and they rarely struggle with just one.

1. Guilt
2. Embarrassment
3. Inability to identify help
4. Fear of asking for help and being refused
5. The person(s) helping "may do it wrong" and create a bigger mess
6. The person(s) helping may abandon the caregiver

Regardless of why we won't ask for help, it doesn't negate our need.

What happens to the individual(s) depending upon you if you go down physically, fiscally, or emotionally? How will that vulnerable person function if extreme stress and weariness impair your judgment?

Asking for help is not a sign of weakness or defeat but rather one of wisdom—and is usually accompanied by humility and a bit of faith. The phone may feel like it weighs 100 pounds in those moments, but the rewards far outweigh the risks. The benefits of accepting help extend beyond assistance with tasks. Receiving support connects us to the strength and love of others— all of which better fortify us for the long journey of caregiving.

● ● ●

It is not so much our friends' help that
helps us, as the confidence of their help.
—Epicurus

83

Get Used to Ambiguity

• • • • •

When expressing frustration at the lack of answers and a clear path through caregiving challenges, a friend told me, "Get used to ambiguity."

For many caregivers, closure remains elusive until after a funeral—and tenuous even then. While solutions, answers, and definitive courses of action seem luxuries often denied to caregivers, demanding to know why and how seems hardwired into not only our emotional DNA, but also our culture's.

During the first six months of the pandemic, try to count how many advertisers used the phrase, "During these uncertain times . . ."

Yet when were times certain?

Ambiguity exists all around us—not as chaos but as things beyond our control. Making peace with things we can't control helps us see that most of the confusion and disorder we rage against comes from within. Recently faced with another of those circumstances, I recalled my friend's counsel and chose to shake hands with ambiguity—again. While doing so doesn't remove the journey's discomfort and weariness, it makes it less rocky and stressful.

• • •

Man lives in a world of surmise, of mystery, of uncertainties. —John Dewey

84

Anger Management

• • • • •

Dear Peter:

How do I not become so angry? —Leslie, with clenched fists

Dear Leslie:

Sometimes anger is warranted. However, anger directed at an impaired loved one's behavior can be futile. How do you get angry with a disease? In cases where your loved one is behaving poorly and even inappropriately, try to detach from it and realize they're oftentimes not doing it to you—they're just doing it.

When the anger hits you, take a moment to breathe: four seconds in, eight seconds out. Drink some water, take a walk, and practice responding, not reacting. As a cautionary note, anger differs from rage in that rage usually comes from a place of great fear—or wounds. If you find yourself raging out, seek professional help immediately. Ask a clergy member or primary care physician to recommend an appropriate counselor.

Your peace of mind is just that: yours. No one can take it from you, but you do have the power to give it away.

• • •

Anger is an acid that can do more harm
to the vessel in which it is stored than
to anything on which it is poured.
—Mark Twain

85

Waffles and Well-Being

· · · · ·

From extended hospital stays surrounded by faceless people in masks to longer nights where loneliness and fear serve as companions, caregivers remain prone to feeling adrift and disconnected.

Longing for recognizable landmarks that signal safe harbor, caregivers face the challenge of "re-anchoring" themselves—often in a storm. But it doesn't have to be complicated. During my wife's surgeries in Denver, I stepped into a Waffle House near the hospital. I love Waffle House. I grew up going to Waffle House, but we now live in Montana, and there's no Waffle House in the whole state!

In Denver, where I knew few people, everything required learning and adjusting. But stepping into the local Waffle House, familiar sounds, sights, smells, and tastes flooded over me. For a few minutes, I reconnected and felt at home. Grabbing a take-out order, I took it to the hospital to share "the familiar" with Gracie.

While we can't always change the disorienting circumstances we find ourselves in, we can find new ways to connect to things that settle our hearts. Sometimes, it's as simple as a waffle—with pecans (and chocolate chips for Gracie!)

● ● ●

I have always loved Waffle House.
It's been like an oasis in the desert many
times late at night after one of my concerts.
—Trace Adkins

86

"Board Certified in What?!"

* * * * *

Due to my wife's early morning surgery schedule, her surgeon instructed me to enter through the emergency room to be with her before the operation.

Approaching the security desk at the ER, I provided my wife's name and shared, "I'm here for her operation."

Verifying her name, the guard stated, "You must use the front entrance."

"It's closed. The surgeon told me to come here."

"You have to use the front entrance," she repeated.

"It's closed. The surgeon me directed here," I restated slower.

The guard repeated herself.

This time I asked, "Where did I lose you?"

A lifetime as a caregiver in more than a dozen hospitals, I've encountered plenty of clipboard-carrying "Barney Fife" types.

"Ma'am, I am board-certified in cranial proctology. They called me from pre-op—I need to be there now!"

Her eyes widened as she waved me through. Smiling to myself, I arrived in pre-op in time.

While cranial proctology isn't an in-demand specialty (except in Washington, DC), I laughingly tell others that I've developed an expertise and use it to help with bureaucratic roadblocks. With a bit of creativity and a poker face, caregivers can often navigate those roadblocks and "clipboard carriers" without adding more drama to our already challenging life.

● ● ●

"I ain't got time to stand around here and discuss trivial trivialities." —Barney Fife,
The Andy Griffith Show

87

If It's Hysterical,
It's Historical

• • • • •

Think back on an encounter with an adult overreacting to a situation. Were you caught off-guard? Did you feel uncomfortable? A psychiatrist friend of mine shared a phrase he often communicated to his staff: "When you see a patient overreact or act out, always remember there's a story behind that behavior."

Adults don't lose self-control in a vacuum—there's a build-up and a story behind their behavior. When caregivers find themselves in the unpleasant predicament of engaging an individual with frenetic or hyper behavior, it's helpful to remember that the behavior is more significant than the moment.

Reminding ourselves that "there's a story" enables us to speak to the deeper issues driving the outburst—which often requires assurance rather than reason. Arguing with a longtime wound is futile. Caring for that wound and its symptoms remains a more effective response. As caregivers, we encounter those panicking about pocket-sized problems. Outbursts at a temporary or minor problem are rooted in a long journey that could stretch back a lifetime. Detaching from the immediate eruption allows us to understand better and address the volcanic turbulence behind the explosion.

However, it starts with us remembering, "If it's hysterical, it's historical."

• • •

We are not makers of history. We are made
by history. —Martin Luther King Jr.

88

Respecting the Trauma

• • • • •

Let's face it; many people don't know what to say when encountering someone struggling with divorce, broken relationships, a tragedy, or other painful realities. In sincerity, some offer suggestions like:

That's in the past. Just put it behind you. Don't look in the rearview mirror.

While sounding like good advice to keep moving forward, there are times when acknowledging the magnitude of someone's heartache is appropriate— and "sifting through the mess" and assessing the destruction is required. Recovery takes time, and part of the process involves meticulously inspecting the damage. Any insurance adjuster who's visited a client following a devastating flood, fire, or tornado will affirm the importance of an exhaustive appraisal of the damage before rebuilding.

Many caregivers painfully discover the journey doesn't end at the cemetery. In some instances, the aftereffects of caregiving can last a lifetime. All too many caregivers can attest to the lasting impact of caring for an impaired loved one, and more studies are needed to show the PTSD statistics of family caregivers.

Trained professionals and loving family and friends can help caregivers navigate a path to healing. However, the first step always involves thoroughly inspecting—and respecting—the trauma.

• • •

We've got to rebuild human hearts—and persuade people that hope isn't just possible, but essential. —Tony Snow

89

Fretting Is Exhausting

· · · · ·

My high school chemistry teacher's name was, no kidding, Mr. Faile. While a hilarious and exceptional teacher, he made the dreaded (for some) class even more daunting by posting a sign over the chalkboard that read, "Flunk Now and Avoid the Rush."

For those born after 1980, a chalkboard was an ancient education device that doubled as a screeching torture machine.

That sign still sticks with me, and I've appropriated the message into other areas of my life—particularly as a caregiver. Accepting reality and not delaying the inevitable becomes a path of wisdom rather than a depressing conclusion. As caregivers, we place unreasonable demands on ourselves to achieve or alter things we cannot change.

Despite extensive striving and colossal anxiety, caregivers will inevitably "flunk" at changing most of what we worry over. Embracing that premise allows greater peace of mind today.

I passed high school chemistry (barely), but Mr. Faile's most important lesson to me had nothing to do with formulas and equations. A simple sign meant in jest communicated a greater truth that still helps bleed off stress—a lifetime later.

Rest now and avoid the crash. We face challenges better when not exhausted by fretting.

• • •

The pitcher has got only a ball. I've got a bat. So the percentage in weapons is in my favor and I let the fellow with the ball do the fretting. —Hank Aaron

90

An Instant Vacation

· · · · ·

Legendary comedian Milton Berle ("Mr. Television") once stated, "Laughter is an instant vacation." Caregivers certainly top the list of those needing an "instant vacation," but few permit themselves to book the trip. A caregiver's life remains full of harsh realities that seemingly eradicate even a chuckle.

Certainly, humor's not something you can experience as a caregiver—or is it? The challenge for all of us is to learn to use humor as we would any other tool. It takes practice, skill, and the belief that life can be lived with gusto, even in challenging situations. I've played the piano for hundreds of funerals and witnessed countless times where humor helped the healing process of loss. Sorrow and pain remain unavoidable, but joy and a sense of humor are choices. Of course, one doesn't want to be clueless and unable to "read the room," but we can enter any room knowing that all life is beautiful—and there is a place for laughter.

Maybe today is the day to take an instant vacation and allow some laughter—even for a moment. If unclear where to start, try *The Three Stooges*—they always work for me! *"Nyuk, Nyuk, Nyuk!"*

● ● ●

Laughter is the sun that drives winter from the human face. —Victor Hugo

91

Stock Answers

• • • • •

A friend recently shared the challenges he and his wife currently face with breast cancer. Relaying the journey through chemo and other issues, I could tell that, while strong, they both carried great apprehension. Knowing my long journey as a caregiver, we chatted about various experiences and tips, and then I surprised them with an odd suggestion. "It's okay to have stock answers."

Tilting their heads, I explained that although many people may ask about their challenges, most people cannot process the reality of their journey. "They want to be polite—and they sincerely care, but it doesn't mean you must bare your soul to everyone who asks."

Stock answers aren't shallow or trivial; they are tools to communicate enough information to those not closely connected.

She's not where she'd like to be, but she's improving.

He's had a rough go recently, but his spirit is strong.

She's a bit overwhelmed but hanging tough—thank you so much for asking.

People do care—and they want to express that concern. However, caregivers can easily overshare and inadvertently push others away. The deep feelings and intimate details are best saved for a close circle of friends, family, support group, or counselor.

• • •

"Thank you for caring" is a complete
sentence. —I coined this

92

Staying in Our Lane

· · · · ·

Although caregivers don't monopolize frenetic behavior, our struggle with freaking out seems disproportionate. While yearning for the open road where we can ease into cruise control, we mostly find ourselves in stop-and-go traffic—watching the needle on our RPMs continually hitting the redline. Staying with the traffic analogy, we often slam our fists on the steering wheel while craning our necks to find a better lane.

What if there's no better lane? Can we make peace with where we are—and somehow be content?

While the short answer is "yes," that path is often rejected due to fear, the clock, guilt, resentment, and other issues. The hard truth is that the crucible of caregiving keeps us in a place where we must either accept limitations—or live with an unbearable (and unsustainable) level of agitation.

Yet when embraced, even hard truth arrives with a reward. Wisdom, peace, and maturity always accompany decisions to accept an unchangeable circumstance. Such acceptance results in frenzied behavior dissipating and a lot fewer RPMs on our hearts.

• • •

*Bless you, prison; bless you for being in my
life. For there, lying upon the rotting prison
straw, I came to realize that the object of life
is not prosperity as we are made to believe,
but the maturity of the human soul.*
—Aleksandr I. Solzhenitsyn

93

Work the Problem,
Fly the Plane

●　●　●　●　●

Several pilots I know express a standard command often given to less experienced pilots.

"Work the problem and fly the plane."

The context involves pilots who fixate on a problem like a storm, console light, or other issues. Riveting one's eyes on a single point to the exclusion of the bigger picture can quickly result in disastrous outcomes—particularly when piloting an aircraft.

Locking in on one issue while dangerously losing perspective is not exclusive to pilots. Caregivers frequently spiral out of control while arguing with an impairment like Alzheimer's disease, alcoholism, or addiction—all of which easily overpower a caregiver and divert eyes from "flying the plane."

Our responsibility as caregivers is to see the bigger picture when our loved ones can't. Just like every passenger in the plane depends on the pilot not losing focus, so do all who rely upon us as caregivers.

While no one would think of handing over a plane to an untrained individual, caregiving sadly serves as the ultimate "on-the-job training" environment. Even the best of caregivers discover they are outmatched and ill-prepared. That's why each of us requires regular reminders to keep calm and "work the problem and fly the plane."

• • •

Let your eyes look directly forward,
and your gaze be straight before you.
—Proverbs 4:25 ESV

94

The Secret of Triumph

· · · · ·

A car accident many years ago left a former coworker with significant bone loss in her leg that led to a terrible walking gait for more than twenty-five years. However, one day, she arrived at the office looking like a different person. Standing straight and walking with no limp due to an orthotic shoe with a lift, we all expressed astonishment at the transformation.

Three weeks later, however, she limped back into the office. Asking her what happened, she responded, "It was too painful to change."

For a quarter of a century, her muscles and tendons adapted to her injuries and limp. Retraining her body proved intensely uncomfortable – and she reverted to the familiar.

Her sad story mirrors so many of ours. Sometimes, injuries cripple us significantly, and even with adaptive help, retraining our wounded hearts and souls is so painful that we give up. Although challenging, change is possible—but it often requires us to dig deep. Supportive friends, families, and trained professionals are critical—particularly during the early stages.

The first day my wife walked on two prosthetic legs, I cheered her on as she took ten painful steps across the room to her prosthetist.

The next day, she took more.

Like Gracie, each positive step we take with our wounded souls is a victory.

• • •

Perseverance, secret of all triumphs.
—Victor Hugo

95

Know Your Jurisdiction

· · · · ·

In the 1985 Western *Silverado*, Sheriff John Langston (played by John Cleese) obligingly led a posse after two brothers following the breakout of one from the town jail. While chasing the men (whose crimes were questionable), the posse rounded a bend to unexpected gunfire from one of the brothers' companions. As his deputy urged them to push on by yelling, "They're almost out of our jurisdiction," a bullet clipped the sheriff's hat and sent it flying.

Wheeling his horse around, Cleese stated in his wonderfully clipped British accent, "Today, my jurisdiction ends here!"

Returning to town, Sheriff Langston lived to fight another day.

Sometimes, our jurisdiction as caregivers requires reassessing. Many can recall feeling pressure (either from others or ourselves) to "right a wrong," seek satisfaction, or try to force an issue. Yet that pressure can lead us outside our scope of responsibility. Leaving our territory can easily result in unpleasant circumstances—for us, our loved ones, and others.

The temptation to chase after the "ones that got away" can sometimes feel compulsory. In those moments, we serve ourselves well by asking, "How important is this?"

Addressing that question helps reestablish our jurisdiction—and can allow us to fight another day.

● ● ●

He who conquers himself is
the mightiest warrior. —Confucius

96

The Small Victories

· · · · ·

"Wins" come in many forms and serve as important milestones to those fighting impossible odds. Although temptation beckons for us to fix issues that aren't ours, or fear shouts at us to fight something we can't beat, the small victories over things within our immediate ability build confidence—and security. Even minuscule achievements during a storm help establish a beachhead of normalcy and success.

In the movie *We Were Soldiers*, Mel Gibson's character, Col. Hal Moore, stood under massive enemy fire in Vietnam and barked simple orders to the frightened young men under his command.

"Take that creek bed!"

Relying on their training and focusing on the straightforward task of taking a creek bed equipped the soldiers to transcend their fear. The objective became clear, and further goals would present themselves following incremental accomplishments.

While those soldiers faced more brutal circumstances than most, our fear and disorientation are no less real. Small wins warrant respect in the face of crushing odds that so many caregivers endure.

Victories, however tiny, define our progress—not our pace.

• • •

Celebrate even small victories.
—H. Jackson Brown Jr.

97

Journey to the Sunset

· · · · ·

Many families struggle with a loved one facing encroaching cognitive impairments—and the decision points serve as heartbreaking reminders of life's fragility. Sometimes, the impaired loved one seems "normal," yet those moments only serve to confuse caregivers.

"He seemed okay today."

"Mom appeared to rally."

But he's not okay. Mom's not rallying.

The "valley of the shadow of death" can be agonizingly long and painful for some, and it's particularly heartbreaking to watch the decline of those who loomed large in our lives.

Yet, all is not gloom or loss. The wave of sadness initially causes many to panic and fight against the sense of drowning. With help, work, faith, and often a sense of humor, family caregivers in these circumstances can achieve the often-elusive peace of mind—and the more significant conquest of experiencing beauty in the heartache.

Leaving the stage does not mean defeat nor end the zest for life and accomplishment. Dylan Thomas urged this when writing to his father, "Do not go gentle into that good night."

We fight until the end—not to avoid death but to fully embrace life.

• • •

I now begin the journey that will lead me into the sunset of my life. —Ronald Reagan, following his Alzheimer's diagnosis

98

The Box of Things Requiring Redemption

• • • • •

A demoralizing point for many family caregivers lies in unmet expectations, hopes, and dreams. We often visualize what could be—but things beyond our control are roadblocks. Ashamedly, I admit to attempting control and trying to force things on more than one occasion—only to frustrate myself, my wife, and (many) others. Letting go of those hopes and expectations, however, can be painful. Over the last few years, I've tried a different approach. In my mind, I envision a rather large container I call "The Box of Things That God Will Have to Redeem."

Offloading those items, losses, heartaches, and disappointment to God reduces my angst and the potential for resentment.

For me, the box is genuine and reflects my faith that God will indeed redeem each of those things— He's better at carrying them than me. Saying that "God will have to redeem" does not demand the

Almighty to act; it simply recognizes that He alone has the power to do so. Of course, the temptation to retrieve items and stew on them often grips me. Yet I can affirm each time I place them back in the box, I grow less tempted to dwell on them.

After decades of trying to carry the impossible, I find I breathe easier and live more peacefully when trusting God with all the broken pieces. Remembering Jesus was a carpenter further bolsters my faith—knowing He doesn't even waste the sawdust.

• • •

And God shall wipe away all tears from
their eyes; and there shall be no more death,
neither sorrow, nor crying, neither shall there
be any more pain: for the former things are
passed away. —Revelation 21:4 KJV

99

The Calling for Each of Us

• • • • •

Dear Peter:

> I've been caring for several family members, and there's no end in sight. Is Caregiving my calling? —Theresa, questioning her skill sets

Dear Theresa:

> Your calling implies an authority outside yourself that speaks to your purpose. I can't answer whether God has called you to this. Yet here you are, and I am convinced you can function in this role. Furthermore, I am equally confident that God can, and will, continue to equip you to travel this journey.

> Caregivers often feel thrust into something that overwhelms us, and we feel discouraged when we fail. Just because you make mistakes along the journey doesn't disqualify you from the task.

Loving another human being is the calling for each of us.

Sometimes that love requires care, commitment, and self-sacrifice that seems disproportionate to others. As we do this, however, we soon learn that while we may not feel adequate or suitable for it, we discover we can be better individuals through this.

Being better in it brings the benefit of loving deeper, appreciating beauty more profoundly, and walking calmer in storms and challenges.

Even if you don't feel that it's your specific calling, that's a calling worthy of answering.

• • •

There is no greater calling than to serve your fellow men. There is no greater contribution than to help the weak. There is no greater satisfaction than to have done it well.
—Walter Reuther

100

Perception Isn't Always Reality

• • • • •

While in Ghana with our prosthetic limb outreach, *Standing With Hope*, Gracie and I visited a church in the port city of Tema. Following the service, I met a tall, impressive man wearing a flowing white traditional costume with gold trim. With a thick English/Ghanian accent, I heard him introduce himself as "de King, Amos."

Never meeting a king, I felt a bit tongue-tied and stammered, "Sir, I apologize—I don't know how to properly address you."

With a huge smile, he offered in his deep voice, "Just call me "Amos."

"Sir, I can't just call you that," I replied, but he graciously continued chatting. Shortly after, while attending a reception with the pastor, I exclaimed, "I just met the king!"

With a perplexed look, the pastor asked, "What king?"

"The king, Amos," I replied.

Thinking for a minute, the pastor exploded in laughter and spoke in his native language to the room full of Ghanaians who also started chuckling.

Sheepishly, I asked him to explain.

With his equally thick Ghanian accent, the pastor laughed and shared. "You met a church officer, 'Deacon' Amos—not 'De King,' Amos."

Perceptions often cloud hearing. The man looked regal, and perception allowed my ears to misinterpret. While my mistake only resulted in laughter, many misconstrued conversations can result in hurt feelings, resentment, and fractured relationships.

Caregiving breeds isolation, and isolation distorts perception—which leads to significant challenges. Asking for clarification, regardless of embarrassment, always trumps misunderstanding.

● ● ●

Studies have shown that 90% of error in
thinking is due to error in perception.
—*Edward de Bono*

101

"It's the Least We Can Do!"

· · · · ·

Despite carefully booking the appropriate handicapped-accessible room, we arrived in Denver earlier this year for Gracie's surgery only to have the wrong disability accommodations at the hotel. Exhausted, we made the best of it, and since the hospital admitted Gracie the next day, we pushed the inconvenience to the back burner.

Remaining in that hotel following her surgery, I broached the topic with the night manager late one evening—who sincerely apologized for the mishap. Looking at the Ramen soup I was purchasing, she earnestly offered, "Here, take this on us—it's the least we can do."

Summoning a surprising level of self-control, I suppressed the urge to retort, "Of course, it's the least you can do; it's Ramen soup—there's nothing 'least-er'!!"

Restrained by her sincerity, I thanked her for her graciousness and left to relive my college days by quietly fixing Ramen soup while laughing at her absurd remark. Although pushing back may have resulted in financial satisfaction (and possibly a second serving of soup), I let it go and enjoyed a peaceful evening instead. Checking out several days later, the day manager asked about my stay. Better rested, I used that opportunity to address the issue. The manager promptly rectified the mistake in dollars rather than soup.

When weary, sometimes it's best to hold your tongue, enjoy a private laugh, and maybe even have a bowl of soup.

• • •

Give thy thoughts no tongue.
—William Shakespeare

102

Extra Space and Support

• • • • •

I recently returned to the doctor to seek additional help with my left foot's ongoing and vexing problem. Patiently pointing out where my arch was falling, he identified the culprit as an "excessive number of birthdays."

Showing me a shoe insert he uses, he said, "Your days of walking barefoot or wearing shoes without arch supports are over. Get the support you need—and then get a wider shoe."

Following his orders, I ordered the inserts he recommended for my boots and a new pair of broader sneakers. Extra support and more space seem to be doing the trick.

Despite now possessing several pairs of shoes that will be dropped off at the "Nearly New," I learned an excellent principle for family caregivers.

We benefit from the extra support of family, friends, doctors, counselors, and clergy - and we desperately need space from toxic individuals who criticize or even those who consume our time white-boarding solutions like, "Have you tried this? What about doing this?"

While many yearn for "big victories," sometimes the win for caregivers can be a less painful walk through the often drama-filled caregiving journey.

Relationships, like shoes, aren't worth much if they're painful.

• • •

If the shoe fits, wear it. —Unknown

103

An Escape Plan from Mania

• • • • •

Dear Peter:

Why does my mother go through bouts of mania? —Ramona, feeling overwhelmed

Dear Ramona:

Mania stems from a variety of sources. Some psychological, some physiological. Step one is to make sure your loved one's physician is aware of this behavior—and ask for an action plan. It's a good idea to avoid arguing or debating the behavior with your loved one. Trying to reason with manic behavior will only compound the problem and frustrate both of you.

With proper treatment from physicians, manic behavior can be addressed. When that behavior is directed at you, try to detach from it. Realize an illness is attacking you, not the person. Having escape plans for your heart (and sometimes for you physically) can keep you from becoming embroiled in the manic behavior. As caregivers, the more we educate ourselves regarding our loved one's condition, the better equipped we become to endure it—and avoid some of the landmines and triggers.

• • •

Manic depressive is a disease.
—Debbie Reynolds

104

"Let Me Be Brutally Honest"

· · · · ·

A recent article listed annoying phrases permeating our culture's conversation. Statements like, "I'm sorry if I offended you" or "At the end of the day," were, of course, included—but an additional phrase buried in the list captured my attention:

"Let me be brutally honest."

Most at the receiving end of that phrase can affirm that what follows leans more toward brutal rather than honest.

Like a fighter adjusting an opponent's chin to deliver a knockout punch, "let me be brutally honest" is often a setup to a haymaker. Those who lead with that phrase are not asking for consent. And it's doubtful they will accept "no" before charging ahead. Furthermore, while honesty often requires discretion, it does not need permission.

And who wants to allow brutal treatment?

Hearing that phrase from others is bad enough, but how many caregivers speak brutally honest with themselves—to rebuke rather than reform?

Candid conversations offer clarity of circumstances without the berating. "Despite my mistakes, here's what's working and what can improve."

Constructive words and a softer tone (with others and ourselves) won't absolve failures and missteps but can promote a more honest evaluation—minus the brutality.

● ● ●

The person who is brutally honest enjoys
the brutality quite as much as the honesty.
Possibly more. —Richard J. Needham

105

The Comfort of Gratitude

· · · · ·

Resentment can lead even the best of hearts into poor judgment, wrath, and even self-destruction. For caregivers, the fight against bitterness remains perpetual. Maybe family and friends left us out to dry, a bad medical call, an employer fired us in a vulnerable moment, or a drunk driver who caused incalculable pain—there seems no end to the opportunities to hold a grudge. Some caregivers even resent themselves, while others shake their fists at God.

Regardless of the resentment's object, the one who carries the hatred pays the highest price.

The only antidote to the poison of resentment is gratitude—what Cicero called the "virtue from which all others spring." Gratitude always leads to peace of mind, but bitterness only swindles serenity by deceitfully making us feel powerful in our wounded hearts.

Thanksgiving is not simply a meal—nor even a holiday; it's a way of life that refuses resentment's tyrannical hold on our souls.

While incurred wounds are real and painful, they can only fester when we nurse them with the septic cloth of resentment. Thankfulness washes those wounds clean and allows them to heal.

• • •

The soul that gives thanks can find
comfort in everything; the soul that
complains can find comfort in nothing.
—Hannah Whitall Smith

106

Seeing the Helpers

· · · · ·

Discussing recent chaotic events, a woman recently threw up her hands in exasperation over caring for a loved one with mental health issues.

"We could have had her institutionalized and created buffers, but her psychiatrist at the time felt it would be too traumatic for her," she sighed wearily.

After listening, I asked, "How long before *your* trauma surpasses the possible trauma suggested by the psychiatrist?

Friends, family, and even medical providers often underestimate the trauma incurred by family caregivers. Caregiving stress can lead to health issues such as high blood pressure, depression, alcoholism, and binge eating. Not stopping with the body, caregiving stress also attacks the wallet, careers, and relationships—and can even involve emotional and physical abuse.

How many care plans for the chronically impaired presume upon the labor of the family caregiver? Responsible physicians would undoubtedly recognize a morbidly obese caregiver pushing a patient's wheel-chair. Can emotional distress be noticed with the same ease?

Following our discussion, this woman purposed to work with her relative's new psychiatrist and advocate for herself and other family members—not just the one with the mental health issues. Although often overlooked, the trauma to the caregiver always affects at least two lives.

• • •

When I was a boy and I would see scary things in the news, my mother would say to me, "Look for the helpers. You will always find people who are helping." —Fred Rogers

107

Nostalgia Isn't Everything It Used to Be

• • • • •

How many caregivers put themselves through unnecessary stress trying to re-create Christmas traditions?

While a tree, decorations, meals, and gifts remain important, too many allow trappings to eclipse the season's meaning. Sometimes the fear that this may be our loved one's last Christmas pushes us to ensure everything is perfect. But what have we accomplished if we're exhausted or even resentful by December 26?

One of the great joys I've experienced by living in Montana is the opportunity to slow down. When we lived in Nashville, it seemed we raced around at breakneck speeds. The Christmas season there seemed frenetic on a good day. Here in Madison County, I am learning to move at the pace of the weather, the people, and the odd deer, elk, or cow on the road.

If, as Andy Williams so spectacularly sang, "it's the most wonderful time of the year," should we not savor Christmas rather than suffer through it?

The decorations don't have to look like last year's. The menu may change, and the gifts may be more personal than opulent. The time we spend with one another and reflecting on the season's meaning brings more value than our labors or purchasing powers. Nostalgia doesn't spread Christmas cheer—hearts do.

● ● ●

May we not "spend" Christmas
or "observe" Christmas, but rather "keep" it.
—Rev. Peter Marshall

108

An Instrument of Peace

• • • • •

Walter Kirchhoff stepped into history on Christmas Eve in 1914 when the opera singer/German officer sang *"Silent Night"* in both English and German on the battlefields of World War I. On a "beautiful moon-lit night, frost on the ground," Kirchhoff's voice rose from the trenches—and touched battle-hardened soldiers from Belgium, France, Germany, and England. The moment's poignancy spurred other soldiers to sing while temporarily laying down arms. Incredulously, the battlefield became festive as soldiers tentatively walked toward one another and extended Christmas greetings. Despite Pope Benedict XV's earlier plea for a Christmas truce, the fighting had continued until soldiers chose to sing rather than shoot.

Kirchhoff, more than likely, had no idea of the resulting impact of his voice echoing over the scarred landscape; he followed his heart and honored the moment. Sadly, the truce was temporary. Yet, history doesn't record the first soldier to resume firing; it only remembers the one who first sang of peace, reverence, and the meaning of Christmas.

The teachable moment extends today. Families remain filled with conflict over caregiving challenges—many of which may erupt at Christmas gatherings. Yet the precedent stands: in the darkest of times, one voice lifted heavenward can calm a battlefield.

If enough follow Kirchhoff's example, we might not only witness a truce—we may also have peace.

• • •

Lord, make me an instrument of Thy peace.
Where there is hatred, let me sow love.
—St. Francis of Assisi

109

Serenity Now!

· · · · ·

While baseball historically served as America's national pastime, outrage (and mostly rage) now seems the predominant activity. Turning off television, radio, and social media certainly helps disconnect us from enragement or "out"-rage, but what about the "in"-rage?

How many hearts feel the resentment of unsettled emotional debts—whether those of others or our own? While seething can erupt in unleashed fury, festering feelings can also turn inward and manifest as depression and despair.

Outrage, anger, and indignation may all contain legitimate roots, but most can cringingly recall times when our reactions overshadowed the infractions of others (or ourselves).

Despite the high drama swirling in a caregiver's life, we are not fated to be angrier than anyone else. Even in unpleasant circumstances, peace, grace, joy, and the power to forgive remain readily available to us—but not from yelling out "Serenity Now!" like Frank Costanza in TV's *Seinfeld*.

Although challenges can endure beyond our control, contentment remains a choice.

Berating one another or ourselves is exhausting. Outrage may fuel the media and characterize our national discourse, but we still maintain a choice on whether it defines us as individuals.

• • •

I know what it is to be in need, and I know
what it is to have plenty. I have learned
the secret of being content in any and every
situation, whether well fed or hungry,
whether living in plenty or in want. I can do
all this through him who gives me strength.
—Philippians 4:12–13 NIV

110

Strength in Winter

$\bullet\ \bullet\ \bullet\ \bullet\ \bullet$

During recent snowstorms and frigid temps, one couldn't help but notice how those unfamiliar with Montana weather behaved.

Some painfully discovered that "4-wheel-drive" doesn't mean "4-wheel-stop." So many became stranded that a friend stated, "People had to make an appointment to get stuck."

Caregiving, like the weather, offers no compassion for the unprepared, unaware, and those in a hurry. Yet, the principles used in a good ol' fashioned Montana winter also work for family caregivers: *Slow down, check conditions, inventory needed items*, and *keep emergency plans current.*

With severe weather, most understand hunkering down and riding it out. Yet how many caregivers ignore that principle when dealing with a loved one's chronic impairment? Trying to fight Alzheimer's, autism, or someone's addiction proves as effective as racing through drifts higher than tires or slamming the brakes while cruising on the ice at 60 mph. Even with 4-wheel drive, it won't be pretty.

Like the weather, we also remain powerless over a loved one's afflictions. But how we respond to those conditions affects whether we stay healthier and safer—or wind up in a ditch. Winters bring beauty and inspire hardiness that fosters greater appreciation for the summers. When learning to live peacefully in harsh times, caregivers can likewise discover increased gratitude for respites—and maybe even see beauty along the way.

• • •

In the depth of winter I finally learned
that there was in me an invincible summer.
—Albert Camus

111

Not What We Wish It to Be

· · · · ·

In every case involving a chronic impairment, a caregiver orbits nearby—including for those addicted to alcohol or drugs.

Addicts and alcoholics face only three possible futures: sobered up, locked up (jail or rehab), or covered up (death). For a caregiver in a relationship with an alcoholic or addict, there remains only one healthy path—which always involves boundaries. Addicts are powerless over their addiction—and caregivers are as well. The hardest part of any caregiving journey is accepting one's lack of control of another's dysfunction—and a loved one's addiction only amplifies those feelings. Although most recognize fighting a disease such as Alzheimer's is unwinnable, many feel a significant disconnect in understanding someone's addiction also lies beyond our power. We deceive ourselves if believing we can make someone else change.

We cannot carry the impossible burden of postponing our peace of mind until someone else behaves in a way we want. Acceptance is not approval; even while grieving over another's choices, we can still live more peacefully. Grief indicates acceptance of what is—not what we wish it to be. The path for caregivers of addicts is narrow and often fraught with tears, but it contains the well-worn footprints of countless people who've walked it before.

● ● ●

Acceptance doesn't mean resignation;
it means understanding that something
is what it is and that there's got to be
a way through it. —*Michael J. Fox*

112

Broken Plates

* * * * *

When one spins numerous plates like family care-givers often do, messes are inevitable. Despite the standard of perfection that many caregivers push themselves to achieve, no one ever comes close to accomplishing such a feat—and, similar to that of plate spinners, broken pieces also litter the caregiver's world. For caregivers, those shattered objects look like fractured relationships, arguments, poor health, aberrant behavior, career interruptions, a checkbook on life-support, and in some cases, actually broken dishes.

Despite the inevitable mishaps, caregivers often berate themselves when they occur. One proven way caregivers can recover from things going awry or someone experiencing a meltdown is to remember that not making worse is a victory.

When aiming for the gold medal of perfec-tion, "not making it worse" may seem like a distant silver or even bronze medal, but it's still a victory in the unpredictable world of caregiving. Caring for someone with chronic impairments ensures that a minimum of two flawed and stressed individuals face relentless challenges daily. It's a difficult situation that can quickly spiral out of control. In that context, not making it worse is admirable and worthy of putting a checkmark in the win column. Finish the task, sweep up the broken plates, and shake it off.

● ● ●

You win some, lose some, and wreck some.
—Dale Earnhardt

113

The Answer Is Always No Until You Ask

• • • • •

One of the more challenging aspects caregivers face is asking for help. Because caregiver issues usually don't arrive in a straightforward and orderly manner, many feel tethered to a "whack a mole" game. The anxiety from constant vigilance can disrupt rational thinking and leave caregivers feeling overwhelmed, frenetic, and extremely needy. Then the caregiver usually frets on whether they can relinquish control to someone else—or if the new team member will cause additional problems that require more work to repair. Yet even if identifying the immediate need, caregivers must decide who is the best person to enlist—and determine if that individual will grant their request and offer assistance. However, after all that internal deliberation, embarrassment and fear seem to be the major culprits hindering caregivers from asking for help.

How many caregivers rob themselves of assistance by fearfully questioning, "What if they say no?"

Boldness walks best beside humility, and asking for help often requires (and reveals) remarkable courage.

We can push back on fearing rejection and embarrassment by remembering the answer is always "No" until you ask.

Take a deep breath and ask for help. You may get a "yes."

● ● ●

You do not have, because you do not ask.
—James 4:2 ESV

114

When Happiness Chases Us

• • • • •

In today's angst-driven world, people often commiserate about unhappiness. Many admit feeling miscrable or unsettled due to finances, relationships, health, jobs, or caregiving. Expressing that sentiment, a friend recently lamented, "I'm just not happy."

Instead of asking why, I asked if he felt he was healthy. He seemed puzzled and questioned what I meant. I explained, "Chasing happiness is not a worthwhile goal." Unpacking it further, I shared, "Life has too many ups and downs for us to aspire to happiness constantly. But when we chase healthiness, happiness will chase us. Healthier decisions can be made and achieved all day long, and when our wallets, bodies, relationships, professions, and hearts are healthier, happiness will usually track us down."

When asking someone what makes them happy, many offer vague "pollyanna" responses. However, the answers often get extremely specific when asked what healthier decisions they could immediately make. Whether incorporating boundaries, exercise, making amends, or sticking to a budget, the path to a better life becomes quite evident in the context of healthy decisions.

Even in the crucible of caregiving, we can seek to live healthier lives. In doing so, we discover happiness has a way of sneaking up on us.

* * *

A small behavioral change can also lead to embracing a wider checklist of healthier choices. —Chuck Norris

115

Roll with It

• • • • •

Discussing the impact of his wife getting the flu, I heard a man commiserate, "The whole system shut down." He lamented his plight by referring to housekeeping, meals, laundry, the children, and missed time from work, and their physical relationship.

Asking how long her sickness lasted, he exasperatedly replied, "Four days!"

Calculating internally, I considered I'd logged more than twelve thousand days caring for a wife with significant medical challenges. In a moment of uncharacteristic graciousness, I quietly exited that conversation because I didn't trust my judgment to avoid sarcasm—which would not have been helpful to either of us.

The unfair job description placed on his poor wife notwithstanding, a medical event can indeed derail plans and routines instantly. After recovering from the flu, a family can usually return to the familiar, but with a chronic impairment, "getting back on track" can often prove impossible. One must create a new normal within the abnormal—while gaining the ability to pivot (often on a dime).

Routines remain essential, but in the frequent chaos of caregiving, peace of mind requires flexibility rather than rigidity.

• • •

"Blessed are the flexible for they shall not be bent out of shape." —Anonymous

Conclusion

· · · · ·

At a conference, I once fielded a question from a man who asked how to handle caregiving when the person being cared for doesn't show gratitude. My response was, we're not doing it for their gratitude—we're doing it as a reflection of our character. While this may not have been the answer he desired, it spoke to the core issue of so many caregivers: It's often a one-way street.

It's not that the person we care for is assumed to be ungrateful—some are so impaired they cannot show gratitude. But as caregivers, we must remember we can all give selflessly or even lavishly *on our terms*. Caregiving, however, requires us to provide sacrificially on someone—*or something*—else's terms. Sacrificial giving outside our terms quickly illuminates character defects.

When I set out to talk to fellow caregivers, I bypassed the tips of caregiving (which are plentiful in many greeting cards). I instead focus on the turmoil in the caregiver's heart. That's why I spend more time on resentment, fear, guilt, obligation, despair, and rage than providing information on caregiving tasks.

Gracie and I live with relentless medical challenges, but the relationship principles every couple struggles with still apply to us. Caregiving issues, however dire, don't get to circumvent dignity, courtesy, patience, kindness, and other virtues required in all relationships.

Yet, due to the human condition—our fallibility—caregiving quickly reveals the small reservoir of those needed qualities. That's why we need an inexhaustible source of those virtues—and the grace and courage to make amends when we behave selfishly and poorly.

In my journey as a caregiver, I all too quickly flamed out. My immaturity and poor beliefs about life, love, and God came up short, and I painfully discovered my limitations and character flaws. As others tried to speak to me during my journey, my head understood the words, but those words never made it to my heart.

A missionary friend of mine from college provided wonderful insight into this challenge. He and his wife serve with Wycliffe Bible Translators in the Democratic Republic of Congo, and he mentioned, most in the Congo speak French or Swahili. But when the Scriptures are translated into their tribal tongue—the language of their hearts—that's when "…you see the smiles light up their faces."

One does not translate the Bible on the first day of arriving in a village. It requires years of spending time understanding the culture and lifestyle of the villagers before even the first verse is translated.

I've spent a lifetime immersed in the village of caregivers, and I speak the language fluently. Like my missionary friends, I find my fellow caregivers' faces light up when I communicate to them in a way they understand. While this book represents those efforts to communicate to my fellow caregivers' hearts—the better news is "caregiver" is our Savior's native tongue.

My stewardship of what I have (and continue to learn) is to serve as a crossing guard and help point caregivers to safety—to the one who speaks directly to their broken and wounded hearts.

When referring to Jesus, Scripture states, "He was despised and rejected by men, a man of sorrows and acquainted with grief; and as one from whom men hide their faces he was despised, and we esteemed him not." Isaiah 53:3 (ESV).

That sounds poignantly similar to what many caregivers express they feel in their worst moments.

So, to that man at the conference, and all others, who ask about the lack of gratitude from the one they care for or who feel overpowered by grief and weariness, I use that verse to point to the One who understands sorrow. In doing so, I also point to the One who beckons the weary and heavy laden to come to Him (Matthew 11:28).

My wife has a Savior—I'm not that Savior. I merely serve as a steward while directing her and others to the One who provides grace and strength to endure—even if it's for one minute at a time.

• • •

Now unto him that is able to keep you
from falling, and to present you faultless before
the presence of his glory with exceeding joy.
—Jude 24 KJV

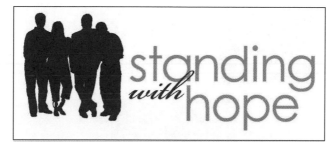

Standing With Hope is the ministry founded by Gracie and Peter Rosenberger. The organization focuses on "the Wounded and Those Who Care for Them" through two programs: a prosthetic limb outreach for amputees and an outreach to family caregivers.

Peter and Gracie invite you to join their mission by visiting standingwithhope.com.

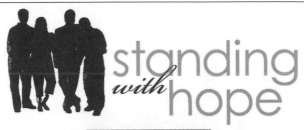

standing *with* hope

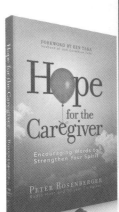

Hope for the Caregiver
Encouraging Words to Strengthen Your Spirit
PETER ROSENBERGER

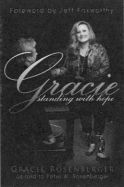

Foreword by Jeff Foxworthy
Gracie
standing with hope
GRACIE ROSENBERGER
as told to Peter W. Rosenberger

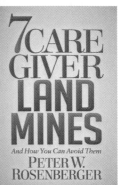

7 CAREGIVER LAND MINES
And How You Can Avoid Them
PETER W. ROSENBERGER

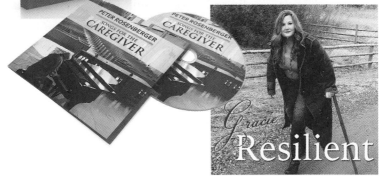

PETER ROSENBERGER
SONGS FOR THE CAREGIVER

Gracie
Resilient